Praise for *Tap, Taste, Heal*

"Many thanks to Marcella for her clarity, compassion, and depth as she takes readers on a comprehensive journey to heal the root causes of body shame and relentless dieting. Marcella supports readers to remove the should's and the shame and replace them with joy and love while living life to the fullest. Let the healing begin!"

—CAROL LOOK, founding EFT master and cocreator of the documentary film *Tapping for Weight Loss*

"As someone who works in the alternative health-care field, I know how important self-care practices are in any healing endeavor. Marcella is a consummate teacher of such practices, and Tap, Taste, Heal *is a great field guide for everyone seeking a self-loving alternative to restrictive dieting and punitive exercise."*

—RENEE RUSSO, founder of the Breast Thermography Center of Sonoma County, California

"I recently met a client of Marcella's who couldn't stop singing her praises. After reading this book, I see why. Marcella's insight and compassion go right to the heart of the issues that people face when struggling with food and body image, and the solutions she offers are life changing."

—KARL DAWSON, founding EFT master, creator of Matrix Reimprinting, and author of *Matrix Reimprinting Using EFT: Rewrite Your Past, Transform Your Future*

"If you use the kitchen only to microwave your 'meals,' let Marcella's Tapping techniques and cooking tips help you learn how to give yourself and others the daily gift of home-cooked food. Marcella has captured so beautifully what it truly means to cook, and this book might well hold the secrets to healing ourselves and our loved ones through the art of home cooking."

—ALMA SCHNEIDER, founder of Take Back the Kitchen: Overcoming the Obstacles to Cooking

"Our beloved natural-foods-chef instructor Marcella taught our students the essence of eating for health—consciously sourced whole foods, lovingly prepared, and eaten mindfully. I'm glad to see her blended wisdom reaching a wider audience with this book."

—ED BAUMAN, founder of Bauman College Holistic Nutrition and Culinary Arts

"Marcella is really insightful and fun. And she really knows her EFT!"

—ROB NELSON, founder of Tapping the Matrix Academy

What Clients Say

"For the first time in my life, I am living free from cravings. This opens up to me a world of choice and fullness that I've never experienced before working with Marcella. Marcella has a surprising ability to pinpoint and help you release exactly what's keeping you stuck. I can now take the energy I used to spend 'fixing' my eating and put it toward things in my life that truly matter to me. I am forever grateful."

—MEREDITH V., San Carlos, California

"Marcella's work is not for the faint of heart. Learning to love myself unconditionally has been gut-wrenchingly hard and beautiful and has required me to dig deep into the most tender parts of my soul. I wanted weight loss, this happened ... but not by counting calories and cutting carbs. It happened because I healed myself from traumas that have been plaguing me for many years. Marcella breathed life back into my soul. I am a work in progress, and I have such immense gratitude for this life-altering journey."

—PAMELA H., Cascade, Colorado

"Working with Marcella was one of the best decisions I've ever made. It was time to face an area of my life that I'd felt beaten by. With Marcella's guidance I have faced the emotional issues behind the weight and feel like I'm actually getting somewhere. I'm losing weight sustainably, I'm coming into right relationship with my body, I feel lighter emotionally and physically, and I'm more confident in my own skin. Marcella's compassionate, loving, wise approach has been a godsend to me. I'm finally getting started on the healing I've desired for years."

—LOLA F., London, UK

"I am so grateful for the series of events that brought me to Marcella. I have embraced many lessons in my work with her, all of which have enhanced my mental, emotional, and physical health, but there have been bigger and deeper lessons along the way. Some required a great deal of self-honesty, soul-searching, and internal struggle. But I wouldn't trade any of these moments if I had them to do over. With guidance and support from Marcella, I have been given the greatest gift of all: I have learned to truly love myself exactly as I am. Oh, and yes, I'm losing weight!"

—CONNIE W., North Myrtle Beach, South Carolina

Tap, *Taste,* *Heal*

Use Emotional Freedom Techniques (EFT) to Eat JOYFULLY and LOVE Your Body

Marcella Friel

Foreword by Rachel Estapa

North Atlantic Books
Berkeley, California

Published by
North Atlantic Books
Berkeley, California

Cover art © Monash/Shutterstock.com
Cover design by Jasmine Hromjak
Book design by Happenstance Type-O-Rama

Printed in the United States of America

Tap, Taste, Heal: Use Emotional Freedom Techniques (EFT) to Eat Joyfully and Love Your Body is sponsored and published by the Society for the Study of Native Arts and Sciences (dba North Atlantic Books), an educational nonprofit based in Berkeley, California, that collaborates with partners to develop cross-cultural perspectives, nurture holistic views of art, science, the humanities, and healing, and seed personal and global transformation by publishing work on the relationship of body, spirit, and nature.

Chapter 8 was previously published in an article in *Elephant Journal,* "Stop Eating Concepts and Start Eating Food." Chapter 9 was originally published in the Tapping Solution Blog, "Breakfast: The Key to a Happy Life."

North Atlantic Books' publications are available through most bookstores. For further information, visit our website at www.northatlanticbooks.com or call 800-733-3000.

MEDICAL DISCLAIMER: The following information is intended for general information purposes only. Individuals should always see their health care provider before administering any suggestions made in this book. Any application of the material set forth in the following pages is at the reader's discretion and is his or her sole responsibility.

Library of Congress Cataloging-in-Publication Data

    Names: Friel, Marcella, 1962– author.
    Title: Tap, taste, heal : use emotional freedom techniques (EFT) to eat
      joyfully and love your body / Marcella Friel.
    Description: Berkeley, California : North Atlantic Books, [2019]
    Identifiers: LCCN 2018048510 | ISBN 9781623173098 (paperback)
    Subjects: LCSH: Emotional Freedom Techniques. | Weight loss—Psychological
      aspects. | Mind and body therapies. | BISAC: HEALTH & FITNESS / Weight
      Loss. | BODY, MIND & SPIRIT / Healing / Energy (Chi Kung, Reiki,
      Polarity). | COOKING / Health & Healing / General.
    Classification: LCC RC489.E45 F75 2019 | DDC 616.89/14—dc23
    LC record available at https://lccn.loc.gov/2018048510

1 2 3 4 5 6 7 8 9 SHERIDAN 24 23 22 21 20 19

Printed on recycled paper

North Atlantic Books is committed to the protection of our environment. We partner with FSC-certified printers using soy-based inks and print on recycled paper whenever possible.

to my mother,

Anna Marrone Friel

(1928–2009)

who always fed me breakfast

and

to Planet Earth,

the mother of us all

Contents

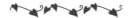

Foreword

WHEN I LOST over sixty pounds several years ago, I was mad that I didn't like myself any better. I felt duped and annoyed that, after months of arduous refinement of what I considered broken—my body—happiness wasn't waiting for me.

Like many women, I spent my youth and early adulthood praying at the altars of dieting. I bought the books and followed the programs, always seduced by effervescent success stories of happy-ever-after once the weight was vanquished. As the number on the scale dropped, I would feel proud and validated. But that fleeting joy was soon followed by exhaustion and anxiety: *how I could keep this up?* There was a gnawing awareness inside of me that to "love myself" went much deeper than trying to change how I looked.

Of course, I was not alone in this struggle. As those of us former chronic dieters know, nearly 98 percent of all diets fail. From as early as age six, we women are indoctrinated to the ever-present message: "Want to be loved? Change your body!" Around the globe, the health and beauty industry makes billions of dollars off women's insecurity about their bodies. Increasingly, we are buffeted by conflicting messages of what we *should* look like—thinner, whiter, younger—in other words, *not how we look right now.* We are taught that the body is separate from the self, and, with the right set of directions, paired with iron will, we should be able to carve a form worthy of approval and praise.

Our bodies are intimately connected to our deepest beliefs about our worth, our value, and our right to be here. So it makes sense that so many of us—especially women—feel like strangers in our own bodies. We're taught that enjoyment comes after sacrifice. That pleasure is only a reward for being good. That happiness is the currency of worth.

When I chose to love my body, whatever its size, I didn't realize just how revolutionary an act it was going to be. Or how hard it would be to shake the web of lies all around me about what my body was allowed to experience. I had to challenge the ideals of beauty, health, and happiness that the fashion industry propagates in mass media and that we've all been indoctrinated to believe. I had to stop hypnotizing myself about what I believed I *didn't* have and shift my focus to what I *did* have. Through this process, I discovered the marvelous truth about my capable body, and I gradually learned that there is *more to love* about myself beyond my appearance.

As part of this process, I challenged myself to try yoga—something I always thought was not made for my body type—and was amazed to find that, when I give my body the support and respect it deserves, yoga is an incredible tool helping me discover and delight in my natural strength, grace, and beauty.

From this deep commitment to myself, I created More to Love, a yoga school devoted to serving the needs of larger bodies. As I've taught thousands the joy of More to Love Yoga, I've not only experienced the life-changing reverberations of a compassionate yoga practice, but I've also reclaimed the broken shards of my past so I could build something better for myself and others.

Fortunately, I'm not alone in my efforts to reclaim dignity, health, and happiness for those of us who occupy bodies larger than what society currently deems acceptable. Marcella Friel, in her thoughtful book *Tap, Taste, Heal,* offers a soothing balm for those of us who have been burned by diet trauma. She not only lovingly holds a compass of kindness for her readers while mapping out a path to unconditional self-love but also provides the tool of EFT Tapping, which readers can use to resolve both immediate and long-term emotional distress relatively quickly and discover the joy that is their birthright.

Often, people confuse self-acceptance with resignation. They believe that to accept means to give up. For some with bodies they are trying to love, acceptance is often equated with failure. They believe that their best efforts to become happy and whole within their body should mean changing it rather than learning to appreciate it. Let *Tap, Taste, Heal* offer you a different concept of self-acceptance as a natural result of healing the traumas that have bound you while opening your eyes to see the beauty, strength, and power of the body you occupy at this very moment.

I know that, after reading and following the exercises Marcella presents in this book, you will come away with a radically different and infinitely more victorious perspective on what loving your whole self really means. I'm so grateful to add *Tap, Taste, Heal* to my collection of works that are profoundly changing the conversation on body love and acceptance, and I look forward to tracking its impact both on your personal life and on the awakening of our new collective body consciousness.

With love,
Rachel Estapa
Founder, More to Love Yoga
Somerville, MA
October 2018

Preface

ON THE MORNING of Monday, October 9, 2017, while visiting my beloved former hometown of Sonoma, California, I woke up to an innocent text from a nearby friend: "Are you okay?"

I had no idea why she would ask me that. Looking out the front window, I saw a typical foggy Northern California morning. Except the fog … was *smoke*.

Something like snowflakes was falling silently from the air.

It was *ash*.

The largest wildfire to date in the history of California was ripping through Sonoma County, burning a few short miles all around me to the north, east, and south. In a few short hours, I saw my homeland of ten years—"God's chosen place on earth," in the words of horticulturalist Luther Burbank—shape-shift from heaven to hell. I was looking straight into the eyes of climate disaster.

As I wended my way through the devastation—helping friends who had lost their homes, evacuating my guest lodging to go who knows where—I continually prayed to the Universe, "Please use me. Let me be helpful in any way I can."

One month later, working in my home office in Southern Colorado, I received an email out of the blue from an old friend and book-publishing colleague of many years, Pamela Berkman, who had recently accepted a position as acquisitions editor at North Atlantic Books in Berkeley. She invited me to submit a proposal to write the book that you are now holding in your hands.

Tap, Taste, Heal is not a book about climate change. It's a book about how to use the remarkably transformative tool of Tapping (also called EFT or Emotional Freedom Techniques) to resolve the myriad conflicting emotions, traumatic memories, and limiting beliefs that drive your struggles with emotional eating, binges and cravings, sugar addiction, and chronic body shaming.

Perhaps it seems to you that these very personal issues have nothing to do with the fate of the planet. In reality, they are directly, intimately, and inextricably connected.

Industrial agriculture—which supplies the fodder for those processed foods we hate to love to eat—is the second-largest emitter of greenhouse gases on the planet. For this and other reasons that I outline in this book, our personal food choices can no longer be exclusively personal. How we eat, what we eat, and, by extension, how we live our lives create impacts that ripple like stones in a pond to our family, our community, our society, the planet, and perhaps even beyond.

So healing our relationship with our food isn't just about us feeling better, though that's certainly a desirable outcome. Mother Earth can no longer finance the dubious luxury of our degraded food choices. It's all hands on deck now. More than at any other time in human history, each of us is needed to manifest the sanity our world so desperately needs, and how can we be sane people if we're not eating sane foods in a sane way?

Beyond Mindful Eating

As eminently aware as I am of the impact our food choices have on this planet, I'm equally aware, after working directly and indirectly with thousands of students and clients, that making sane and health-supportive food choices is far, far easier said than done. In the vast array of techniques available to curb problematic eating behaviors, or any of the myriad diets of the day, the common thread that runs through all of them is the assumption that healing negative food habits *is simply a matter of changing personal behavior.*

Even with the best of intentions, such techniques can engender a subtle stigma of shame and failure within a culture that already brutalizes people for their struggles with food.

While mindful eating is, in fact, indispensable to the healing journey, my experience working with clients and students has shown me that working strictly at the level of behavior ensures that it's only a matter of time until the subconscious mind asserts its agenda and pulls us back to where we believe we belong. In other words, mindfulness and other similar practices, in my experience and my observation, do not resolve the root distress that causes us to soothe ourselves with food to begin with.

In *Tap, Taste, Heal,* I present two core concepts that have helped my clients and students resolve their eating struggles for good:

> *Your struggles with food are not your fault.* A constellation of personal, social, and environmental forces has contributed to the degradation of our collective

eating habits. While you certainly can take responsibility for your healing, it's not your fault you're in this predicament to begin with.

🍃 EFT Tapping is a remarkable tool that can help you resolve the conflicting emotions, traumatic memories, and limiting beliefs that drive your self-soothing food behaviors. When healing occurs at the level of emotions, memories, and beliefs, the behaviors naturally take care of themselves.

Is This Book for You?

While *Tap, Taste, Heal* is not a book exclusively for women, it does speak in a distinctly feminine voice to the people who have sought out my services over the years, 99.9 percent of whom have been women. But as the issues that cause us to struggle with food are, in reality, universal, I do feel that people of all genders, including men, can benefit from the information in these pages.

This book is for you if you suspect that your struggles with food are not entirely about the food. It's for you if you know that restrictive dieting, punitive exercise, and stepping on the scale ten times a day are not the answer. It's for you if you're done with the promise of a quick fix and want to heal these challenges at the root. It's also for you if you don't want one more book that tells you what to eat and what not to eat, but, instead, you want one that addresses and liberates the personal, social, and spiritual roots of your struggles.

Whether you're a big fan of Tapping or are new to the technique, you'll find that *Tap, Taste, Heal* will give you tools you can use right away for both immediate and long-term relief of food behaviors that have plagued you up until now. You might be surprised that something so simple could be so effective.

How to Use This Book

I created *Tap, Taste, Heal* to be both informational and transformational. My intention is to help you develop literacy in the issues that surround your eating problems while giving you this tool of EFT Tapping to resolve them.

With the exception of chapter 1, at the end of each chapter you'll find Tapping guides that are meant to be used like training wheels on a bicycle. As one of the biggest challenges with Tapping is figuring out what to say, I scripted the guides with phrases to give you a jump-start in finding your own words. With Tapping, it's essential always that the words you use resonate with you, and so I encourage you wholeheartedly to use your own words if the ones I've supplied don't hit the spot. Also, for consistency of format, I wrote the guides in verses of four, progressing from the negative to the positive; but again, you might find that your issue isn't fully resolved by the time you get to the fourth round. If that's the case, keep tapping, keep using your own words, and stay focused on the negative as long as you need to. At some point during the tapping you might feel a little "pop" or a shift where the negative emotions no longer have a hold on you. That's the time to start tapping in the positive. The guides are numbered by the chapters they belong to (e.g., 3.1, 3.2, 4.1, etc.), so that you can easily make note of the guides that are particularly helpful to you and find them again at a later date.

I've also provided a Tapping How-to Chart at the end of the book that shows you the points to tap on and summarizes the instructions. Feel free to copy this chart and keep it somewhere handy, to help you entrain yourself to the Tapping process.

Tapping, by nature, is an interactive medium; if you find it challenging to read the Tapping guides and tap along with them at the same time, I've created an online audio Tapping library (and a how-to Tapping video) just for you, dear reader. You can access this library at www.marcellafriel.com/taptasteheal.

Finally, I suggest you keep a journal handy while you read. There are places in the book where I prompt you to answer questions and take notes.

The Journey Ahead

Tap, Taste, Heal begins in part 1 with an introduction to the practice of Tapping in chapter 1, followed by a detailed how-to guide in chapter 2. These chapters will give you the foundation you need to do the Tapping exercises throughout the rest of this book.

Part 2 addresses the most common personal aspects of our struggles with food. If you've tried and failed at restrictive dieting, it's not your fault. I'll show you in chapter 3 how restrictive dieting, in reality, is just a binge waiting to happen.

Chapter 4 takes a refreshingly forgiving look at the whole issue of self-sabotage and shows you that, given what we are up against, your acts of sabotage are not a sign of failure or weakness. They are your soul's way of slowing down progress when it doesn't feel safe to succeed.

Chapters 5 and 6 take a deep dive into the issue of food addiction. In chapter 5 we'll look at the three characteristics of addiction from a twelve-step recovery point of view, and I'll give you the tools you need to heal at each of these levels. In chapter 6 I'll share with you a personal story about the day I gave up my Jackson's Honest potato chips and how it was much more than a snack that I was letting go of. I'll tell you how I did it using Tapping, then guide you through your own process of "Tapping on Your Trigger Foods." You'll never see those foods in the same way again.

Part 2 wraps up with chapter 7, where we get to the heart of the matter: how our limiting beliefs drive our limiting behaviors with food. I'll give you two powerful, effective ways to uncover your core beliefs and walk you through the Tapping techniques that can help you transform *I can't* into *I can.*

Part 3 of *Tap, Taste, Heal* pans the camera away from our personal issues and looks at the broader social context that gave birth to our mindless eating behaviors. In chapter 8 we examine how, historically, we human beings learned what to eat from our traditional foodways and how, in the absence of that wisdom, we have become an unhealthy society obsessed with healthy living. In this chapter I present a fad-proof formula that, combined with Tapping, definitively resolves the vexing question, "What the hell should I eat?"

You've probably heard that breakfast is the most important meal of the day—but have you ever heard *why?* In chapter 9 I'll introduce you to the three key hormones that call the shots on your food behaviors and body weight and show you how a hearty, health-supportive breakfast is the key to keeping those hormones happy and humming. I'll also give you a Tapping guide to use if you feel resistance to nourishing yourself at the start of your day.

In chapter 10 I'll help you transform your kitchen from a dungeon of drudgery to a sanctuary of self-care. We'll talk about what we as a society lost when we stopped eating home-cooked meals, and we'll tap on any "kitchen trauma" you might have, if the prospect of home cooking feels overwhelming to you. You'll also get Chef Marcella's tips and tools for finding creativity and delight in home cooking, whether you're a rank beginner or a seasoned pro.

What would your life—and your food—be like if you could say, "I deeply love and accept myself," and *mean it?* In chapter 11 we'll walk through the all-important terrain of forgiveness, and I'll give you some Tapping tools to help you forgive both yourself and others.

In chapter 12 we celebrate the beauty you are, whatever the scale says. We'll talk about how the fashion industry has instigated and profiteered from our collective body loathing. I'll help you free yourself from that swampland of shame and take you to the mountaintop of unconditional self-love.

In chapter 13 we take a sobering look at food waste and the consequences of super-sized food portions on both the planet and our waistline. I'll then share with you the most powerful ecological tool available right now to reverse this deadly trend on the spot and turn your life into a feast of gratitude.

The final chapter of *Tap, Taste, Heal* will send you on your way with pearls of wisdom about how to embody the success you want to manifest in your life. This chapter includes two powerful guided meditations using EFT to meet your future healed self and to raise your vibration to call in your heart's deepest desires.

I hope you find *Tap, Taste, Heal* as enjoyable to read as I found it to write. I'm so happy and grateful to share this adventure with you and am holding you in my heart with the most profound wish that you find in these pages the healing you desire and deserve. If you'd like to share your experience with me, I'd love to hear from you. Feel free to reach out to me through my website, www.marcellafriel.com. It might take me a while to respond to you, but please know that I've got your back on this.

Peace and many blessings,
Marcella Friel
Crestone, Colorado
September 2018

Acknowledgments

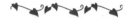

Many times a day I realize how much my own outer and inner life is built upon the labors of my fellow men, both living and dead, and how earnestly I must exert myself in order to give in return as much as I have received.

—ALBERT EINSTEIN

WRITING A BOOK is one of those things that for decades was parked in the back of my brain as a daunting, monumental, "someday-I'm-gonna" project that I imagined would consume my life for years. Were it not for the stalwart faith and unflagging encouragement of my editor and dear old friend Pamela Berkman at North Atlantic Books, *Tap, Taste, Heal* would still be a distant fantasy.

Pam and I met in 1991, in our previous incarnations as editorial staff at a small book-publishing house in San Francisco. Over the years we drew closer and farther away and back again in that double-helix dance that long-term friendships sometimes take, and it's been such a heart-warming delight to discover myself on this side of the editorial equation with her at my side. Pam, you are the Judith Jones to my Julia Child. I love you forever and always.

I also must thank my business mentor and entrepreneurial maverick Dawn Copeland for her unique magic in lifting up my wings, nursing me through squalls of doubt, and always having fearless faith in my capabilities. To the forces of coincidence that brought you into my life, Dawn, I offer thanks and praise.

Mary Sheila Gonnella, the Queen of All Things Nutrition (and the only MSG that's good for your diet), is one of the smartest and kindest women I know. Mary Sheila, it's been so much fun to traipse the yellow-brick road with you, from teaching together at Bauman College in Northern California in 2011 to helping me birth my Women, Food, and Forgiveness Academy. Who knows what's next? Thank you for your sage and savvy *Breakfast Report,* which formed the research basis for much of chapter 9.

When I told my brothers, Howard Friel and John Friel, about this, my first book contract, they both brought me to tears with the sincerity of their joy and celebration. Thanks, you guys, for seeing and holding my success with me. Likewise, I send big love to my sisters, Erin Stone and Patti Durning, for holding the bonds of family through thick and thin. Your little sister loves you back.

When I met Sheila Cataford in the summer of 1987, while in a Buddhist meditation retreat, my first thought was, "She's really cute—I wanna be friends with her!" Little did I know that the Universe would bless us with the fine wine of a spiritual sisterhood that is over thirty years strong and improving with age. Thank you, Sheila, for witnessing, supporting, and celebrating me all these years. Your friendship is pure gold.

A tender thanks goes out to the late Ellen Young, whom I had the privilege of knowing for three too-short years prior to her passing in October 2016. Ellen was my Tapping-training buddy, who swapped endless sessions with me and who taught me, at every stage of her cancer journey, to ask the question, "Can I love myself even with *this?*" Chapter 11 is for you, Ellen.

Big thanks and high-fives also go to Rob Nelson, my EFT mentor and founder of the Tapping the Matrix Academy in Santa Rosa, California, for reviewing chapters 1 and 2 and granting his *nihil obstat* on the content. I'm so grateful we've stayed connected over the years, Rob, and I always appreciate your perspective and support.

Certain of the Tapping guides in this book—namely, "Healing Your Wounded Younger Self" in chapter 7 and "Meeting Your Future Self" in chapter 14—are my adaptations of Karl Dawson's Matrix Reimprinting technique, a genius variation of EFT that is healing the planet one person at a time. I'm deeply indebted to Karl for the profound transformation that his Matrix work has effected in my own life and the lives of my clients.

A deep bow is due to Gary Craig, creator of the EFT technique and keeper of the "Gold Standard" EFT. Gary's altruism and commitment to the highest wellbeing of all have allowed this remarkable tool to spread like wildfire around the globe. Thank you, Gary.

Likewise, I extend deep appreciation to all the thought leaders whose works I reference in this book. Any errors contained in these pages are due strictly to my limited understanding.

A big shout-out is due to local friends who kept me going during the bookwriting process: to my Crestone bestie, Jyoti Stuart, for our healing session swaps and parallel work days punctuated by "civilized lunches"; to Paul, my yoga buddy, who always asked, "How's the book doing, Marcella?" and to Michael, for scooping me up and taking me to soak at the hot springs when the writing became too much. A special thanks too to the Milagros Coffee House in Alamosa, Colorado, for letting me sit, writing away for hours, for the price of a $3 chai latte; and to Nick Chambers and his crew at the Valley Roots Food Hub for all your work on the summer CSA program, keeping me well fed while I wrote. You guys are my local heroes.

I owe deep gratitude to all of my recovery buds over the years, who have kept me sane and sober and remind me always that whatever success I achieve I owe to the God of My Understanding. You all know who you are. I'm so grateful to walk this path with you.

I owe a very special thanks to Madisyn Taylor and the staff at DailyOM (http://dailyom.com) for taking a chance on a brand-new online author and turning my course "Lose Emotional and Physical Weight with Tapping" into a top-ten bestseller. The royalties from that course provided the financial support I needed to create the time that made this book possible. Thank you, Universe, and thank you, DailyOM.

I want to express my delight and gratitude to Rachel Estapa, founder of More to Love Yoga, for blessing my book with her eloquent and heartfelt foreword. Rachel, thanks so much for your generous support. I hope this is the beginning of a fertile collaboration between us.

Thanks are due to Heidi and Tara, the wild and wacky goddesses at In Her Image Photography in Petaluma, California, who can shoot gorgeous images of me while making me laugh so hard that snot runs out of my nose. I don't know how you two do it, but I'm so grateful to you for showing me a beauty within myself that I never knew was possible and for supplying the lovely author image.

Paula Hansen of Chart Magic also deserves a big thanks for creating the Tapping with Marcella chart at the end of this book and putting up with my million-and-one picky-picky changes. You're a trouper, Paula. It's a pleasure to work with you.

Last, I touch my forehead to the lotus feet of the hundreds of clients and thousands of students I've had the deep privilege of supporting over these years. In particular, I owe so much gratitude to the brave heroines in my Women, Food, and Forgiveness Academy who cheered me on with each chapter and reminded me always, "You got this, Goddess Marcella. We love you." Thank you for the privilege of serving all of you. You are the bravest and most beautiful women I know.

–MF

PART 1:

Tap

1

An Introduction to Tapping

IN A WORLD full of failed diet plans, punitive exercise regimens, and countless experts telling us what we're doing wrong, it's easy to believe that our mindless eating habits are hopelessly beyond any possibility of change. But what if those habits could be released with the tap of a finger?

My client Elizabeth knew she had to stop drinking diet soda. What started as a beverage saved for special occasions became an addiction that resulted in soda cases stockpiled in her garage. Having been diagnosed with metabolic syndrome, on medications for clinical depression, and carrying over one hundred pounds of unwanted body weight, she knew the time had come, in her words, to "confront the beast." But the thought of never drinking diet soda again plunged Elizabeth into inconsolable despair.

As she described it, "My relationship with it is incredibly involved. If it's in front of me, I think, 'Let me have it!' If I get upset, it's, 'Where's that diet soda?' When I sit down to a nice meal, the soda better be there to wash it down. It's what I crave to drink. I love the fizzy, sweet, sharp feeling of it, but now it just feels like a mouthful of chemicals. Honestly, it's an assault on my senses. But I can't stop!"

I invited Elizabeth to take a deep breath and reassured her that nobody was going to take her diet soda away, that she got to say when, how, and whether she ever, in fact, let it go. I then guided Elizabeth through some rounds of Tapping in which I encouraged her to lean in to the feelings of deprivation that surfaced at the thought of losing the diet soda. We tapped on phrases such as, "Please don't take away my diet soda," and "No! It's mine! You can't take it away from me!" and "It's the only thing I have that's all mine! I deserve it!"

Right away, with just a few rounds of Tapping, Elizabeth began to feel relief at giving voice to the feelings and thoughts that had been tormenting her. After her initial distress subsided, I invited her to identify her earliest memory of the *emotions* she associated with drinking diet soda.

Together we journeyed back to a six-year-old Elizabeth running away from home, filling a little red wagon with doughnuts to escape the mistreatment she was suffering at her father's hands. While continuing to tap, Elizabeth recalled of her younger self, "She wants to get out—it's not safe—and those doughnuts are the only thing she can rely on. They're her only friend."

With Elizabeth's permission, I guided her through a journey in which she, as her adult self, tapped in her mind's eye on her six-year-old self while reassuring that little one that Daddy's bad behavior wasn't her fault. Tears of relief washed away the dammed-up anxiety Elizabeth had been holding for years. "Wow!" she remarked, "I really can let this go! I feel it! I don't have to carry the guilt over my father's behavior anymore!" Elizabeth wasn't quite sure what the memory of her younger self and the wagon had to do with her diet soda problem, but she did feel immense freedom by the end of our phone call. One week later, she sent me this email:

> Marcella, remember how I said I still felt a little connected to the diet soda at the end of our call? That was due to a feeling of not believing that I could really let go. I had to see it to believe it.
>
> Would you like to know?
>
> I have not had, nor have I wanted, *one diet soda* this week. I have even been in a grocery store and walked right by the mountain-high display of boxes of soda, and it did not have a pull, I just got what I went in the store for, and that was that. No big deal, and no inner dialogue. I have been happy to drink water and mineral water, and my treat drinks have been yerba mate tea, kefir water, and blended water with ice and herbs (basil, parsley, stevia).
>
> So I have to say a miracle has occurred!

Eighteen months later, Elizabeth reached out to me again for more Tapping work. When I asked her about the diet soda, she replied, "What diet soda?" And then she explained, "That's been gone so long I forgot I ever had a problem with it."

What Is Tapping?

Tapping (also called Emotional Freedom Techniques, or EFT) is a gentle, powerful self-help tool that reduces the negative emotional impact of memories and incidents that trigger stress. Some have called Tapping "emotional acupuncture," as it involves fingertip tapping on points at or near the ends of major acupuncture meridians. The tapping disrupts the stress signals that link negative emotions to a particular experience.

Think of it this way: Imagine your dog is barking at the mail carrier. If you just tell the dog to stop barking, what happens? The dog keeps barking. But if you calmly pat the dog on the head and say, "It's okay. It's just the mail carrier; they're not going to hurt us," the dog settles down. This is the basic principle of Tapping. We're literally patting and calming down our "dog brain," which I'll explain in greater detail in just a moment.

There's a saying in the Tapping world: "Try it on everything." EFT can address the whole spectrum of human stress, from minor annoyances to the most profound pain imaginable. I became convinced of the power of Tapping one day when I had lost my keys. I was frantically squawking and pecking about my house, looking for those keys like a despondent mother hen when I suddenly thought, "I can do some Tapping!" After a few rounds, it became crystal clear: I went directly to my gym bag, and *voila!* My keys magically appeared.

Tapping can be extremely effective for working with problematic food behaviors, including

- emotional eating,
- cravings and binges,
- late-night eating,
- eating past being full,
- food allergies, sensitivities, and intolerances, and
- confusion about what and how to eat.

What Do We Mean by "Emotional Freedom"?

Emotions are, literally, *e-motion:* energy in motion. The nature of emotions is that they arise, they dwell, and they dissolve. So *emotional freedom* means a healthy body, brain, and nervous system can allow emotions to flow easily and naturally.

Emotions get stuck when they hook on to an *associative memory.* So let's say, for example, that a stranger walks past you and bumps you in a way that feels aggressive, and you become annoyed. Emotional freedom doesn't mean you shouldn't feel the annoyance, but that the annoyance simply comes up and then moves on.

Now let's imagine that, as that person brushed past you, he made a face that subconsciously reminded you of your father telling you, when you were four years old, that you would never be good enough. That's an associative memory. And when it kicks in, a benign annoyance can flare into a seething rage, and an innocent gesture on the part of a total stranger can ruin your whole day—or even your whole life.

Few things in our lives carry more associative memories than food. That buttery-vanilla-melted-chocolate aroma of Toll House cookies wafting through the downtown bakery transports us back to Big Sister baking batches in the kitchen and the sneaky pleasure of eating them all with her while Mom and Dad were gone. The mere mention of liver and onions churns our stomach as we remember our creepy old uncle with the hairs in his nostrils shoving the plate in our face and saying, "Eat, eat! It's good for you!" And, of course, ice cream—ah, ice cream—and those Friday nights when we had Mom all to ourselves while Dad took the boys bowling, and together we'd cuddle on the couch and plow through a pint of butter pecan while laughing at old movies.

Memories such as these can be heartwarming to recall, but they become deadly when we reach for those same foods years later—except this time it's a gallon of ice cream instead of a scoop—in a subconscious attempt to recreate those feelings of fun, safety, and belonging.

In my client Elizabeth's case, her bondage to diet soda sprang from a subconscious need to hoard food in an infantile attempt to shield herself from Dad's behavior. Somewhere deep in her adult psyche, Dad was still mistreating her, and the doughnuts of her youth (later the diet soda in adulthood) were all she felt she had to soothe herself. It wasn't until that association was broken that Elizabeth's adult perception of the soda as a "mouthful of chemicals" could prevail, and the soda no longer held its addictive lure.

When we tap while recollecting stressful behaviors and their associative memories, as with Elizabeth's diet soda addiction, we send an electromagnetic pulse into our barking-dog brain that lets it know: It's over now. It's just the mail carrier. It's just a diet soda.

What Do We Mean by "Stress"?

Merriam-Webster defines *stress* as "a physical, chemical, or emotional factor that causes bodily or mental tension and may be a factor in disease causation."[1] In human physiology, our ground zero of stress processing is the brain's *limbic system,* where the emotional memorabilia of our life are largely housed. Nestled within our limbic system, on either side of the temporal lobes of our brain, is a tiny almond-shaped section of tissue called the *amygdala*[2] (which is a Greek word for "almond"). The amygdala's job is to scan everything coming in through our sense perceptions and compare it with the memory bank of every bad thing that ever happened to us. If there's a seeming match, whatever it is will register as an imminent danger. When the amygdala perceives a threat (whether real or imagined), it initiates a series of physiological events we've come to know as the *fight-or-flight response.*

One aspect of the fight-or-flight response involves overproduction of a hormone called *cortisol,* which has been linked to various stress-adaptive responses, including sugar cravings, increased appetite, and the development of *visceral adipose tissue* (a.k.a. gut fat).[3]

Cortisol is your best friend when you urgently need to escape a burning building or dodge a car that's swerved into your lane. On a day-to-day level, however, when every email, every deadline, every traffic jam, and every television show feels like that burning building or near car collision, your body's chronic fight-or-flight condition and wild cortisol fluctuations send you, with equal urgency, to that leftover birthday cake in the office break room.

When a stressful experience is especially powerful, the limbic system goes into a kind of hiccup, like a needle skipping on a vinyl record. The associative memory keeps rumbling and recurring in the ground waters of our subconscious until it is interrupted and dispersed neurologically—in this case, by fingertip tapping on points that down-regulate the stress.

The limbic system is also known as the *paleomammalian cortex* and is considered by some researchers to be part of our evolutionary survival adaptation.[4] As such, our limbic system developed in our midbrain millions of years before we developed the more sophisticated upper- and frontal-brain functions of human language and executive reasoning. This is why you can talk about your sugar addiction for years, and you can understand perfectly what it's about and why you're doing it, but that awareness is a booby prize until the problem is resolved at the limbic level.

Is Tapping Just Some New-Age Hoo-Ha?

In 2008, Peta Stapleton, an Australian health psychologist and researcher, conducted a study investigating the effectiveness of EFT for food cravings.[5] Ninety-six obese adults attended a four-week group-based program run by a certified EFT practitioner. The program taught participants how to apply EFT to their feelings and behaviors. The findings showed that EFT had an immediate effect and reduced food cravings. The results were still significant one year later.

The program was then extended to eight weeks, and a clinical trial between 2012 and 2014 compared EFT to the gold standard, Cognitive Behavioral Therapy (CBT), a form of psychotherapy that focuses on modifying negative thoughts, emotions, and behaviors. EFT was proven equally as effective as CBT in increasing restraint ability and power over food, and *superior* to CBT in decreasing food cravings and anxiety symptoms and in maintaining this decrease over one year (in eighty-nine adults).

A Brief History of Tapping

In 1979, Dr. Roger Callahan, a psychologist, began to study traditional Chinese acupuncture and became intrigued by the notion of meridian points and channels as conduits of *chi,* or vital life energy, that run vertically along both sides of the body and are linked to various organs and their functions: the lungs and respiration, the heart and circulation, and so on.

One of Dr. Callahan's patients, who is known as "Mary," was struggling with a phobia of water so severe as to be life threatening. Mary's fear had gotten to the point that simple functions such as bathing and hydration were becoming terrifying.

Dr. Callahan used various psychotherapy techniques with Mary, with no success. With all of his options exhausted, he decided to experiment. Mary complained that every time she thought of water, she got a nervous feeling in the pit of her stomach. Having studied the acupuncture meridians, Dr. Callahan knew that a meridian point directly beneath the eye was connected to the stomach. Not expecting much to happen, he invited Mary to tap lightly on the point beneath her eye. After a few moments, she exclaimed, "It's gone! That horrible feeling I get in the pit of my stomach when I think about water is completely gone!" She leapt up from his office chair and went straight to the edge of his swimming pool, repeating, "It's gone! It's gone!" Her phobia disappeared and never returned.

Shocked and inspired, Dr. Callahan created Thought Field Therapy (TFT), which integrated Western psychotherapy with this new Tapping practice.[6] He developed "algorithms" of Tapping sequences to address different conditions: one for fears, one for anger, and so on. Dr. Callahan began teaching TFT to his students, one of whom was Gary Craig, who discovered it was the tapping itself rather than the somewhat complicated sequences that created the desired results. Gary Craig consolidated Dr. Callahan's algorithms into a single sequence that included all of the major meridian endpoints and that could be used for all issues. Gary named his new technique Emotional Freedom Techniques (EFT).[7]

Feeling passionately that everyone in the world should know EFT, Gary "democratized" Tapping beyond licensed therapists and medical professionals and trained many lay people in this new practice. One of them was Rob Nelson, a psychologist and massage therapist who founded the Tapping the Matrix Academy in Santa Rosa, California, where I was proudly certified as his first graduate.

In the next chapter I will give you instructions on how to begin using Tapping to heal your negative food behaviors.

2

Tapping: The Basic Recipe

DESPITE THE FACT that I've been practicing Tapping for nearly eight years now (as of the writing of this book), and I routinely see legions of my clients and students make quantum shifts in healing their unmindful eating behaviors where other tools have failed, I continue to be gleefully surprised each time I hear about a new breakthrough.

Just this morning, while I was checking in on my students via an online discussion board, Samantha had this to report: "I have noticed some changes, which I might attribute to the Tapping we did in our recent live gathering. I have been serving myself smaller portions of everything and eating less than the entire portion of each thing. Sugar cravings are minimal and infrequent. Tapping is such a great tool!"

Just like playing your first notes on a piano, learning Tapping takes practice. In this chapter I'll walk you through the basic Tapping technique and answer the most common questions people have about this remarkably transformative self-help tool.

Let's Jump In

If you're reading this book, I assume that you've had chronic struggles in your relationship with food that you'd like to resolve at the root, and that you're curious to see how Tapping might help. So let's get started!

Step 1: Focus on the Distress You Want to Relieve

If you have several issues you want to work on, I suggest you focus on what is most stressful in the moment.

Tapping works best when we address our issues as specifically as possible. If, for example, you tap on "I always overeat," you might get some relief, but if you tap on "I eat past the point of being full every night at dinner," you will progress through the issue much more quickly. If you experience multiple issues with food, it's best to address them one by one in separate sessions of Tapping. Here are some suggestions for how specific you can get, taken from my clients' and students' experiences:

- You never eat in front of other people because you feel ashamed of what you eat.
- You feel lonely at night and binge on chips and salty snacks while watching television.
- You overeat when dining out with friends, despite your best attempts not to.
- You're desperate to find a solution to your sugar addiction and feel scared that there might not be one.

Step 2: Assign a Subjective Units of Distress (SUD) Level to the Problem

Once you feel clear on the issue you want to focus on, the next step is to gauge the intensity of the problem using what in the Tapping world we call the *subjective units of distress* (SUD) scale. This is the same 0-to-10 scale a doctor uses when they ask you, "How intense is the pain," with 10 being the most intense and 0 being the least.

If you struggle with finding an exact number, go with how intense the issue *feels* to you in this moment, not how intense you think it should or shouldn't feel.

Making up a list of the issues you're dealing with, arranged from the most stressful to the least stressful, might help you figure out where an individual issue fits on the SUD scale. For the purposes of learning Tapping, I suggest you begin with something that feels like a 5 or higher.

Step 3: Create a Setup Statement

After you know what you want to work on, and you have your SUD level, create what we call the *setup statement*. In the setup statement, you state the problem aloud to yourself and then counter it with a statement of unconditional self-love. Here are some examples of setup statements from the examples of distress I gave earlier:

- "Even though I never eat in front of other people, because I feel ashamed of what I eat, I deeply love and completely accept myself."
- "Even though I feel lonely at night and binge on chips and salty snacks while watching television, I deeply love and completely accept myself."
- "Even though I overeat when dining out with friends, I deeply love and completely accept myself."
- "Even though I'm desperate to find a solution to my sugar addiction, I deeply love and completely accept myself."

While you state the setup statement, you simultaneously tap on the fleshy part of the outside of the hand, where you would hit something or someone with a karate chop. The exact point is about three-quarters of an inch below your pinky, but to make it easy, you can just use all four fingers of your hand to tap the entire side of your other hand. (It doesn't matter which hand taps which.) While tapping on the this point, repeat your setup statement aloud one to three times.

Step 4: Tap around the Points

After tapping on the side of your hand while repeating your setup statement three times, begin tapping lightly on the following eight points, about five to seven times on each point:

1. top of the head (right in the center)
2. inside the eyebrow (where it meets the bridge of the nose)
3. side of the eye (on the bone right in front of the temple)

4. under the eye

5. under the nose

6. under the mouth

7. collarbone point (on either side of the notch of the collarbone)

8. under the arm (commonly referred to as the "bra strap point" on women, about four inches below the armpit)

While you're tapping on the points, say aloud to yourself a short *reminder phrase* to keep the focus on the issue you're tapping on. Again, some reminder phrases from the examples above:

&☙ "This shame I feel ..."

&☙ "This bingeing habit ..."

&☙ "This pattern of overeating ..."

&☙ "This desperation I feel ..."

Do at least one or two rounds of tapping on the sequence of eight points while repeating your reminder phrase. Ideally, continue tapping until you feel a shift.

Step 5: Remeasure Your SUD Level

After you complete a round or two of Tapping, take a deep breath. Revisit your initial distress. How does it feel now? What SUD number would you give it? In most instances, your distress will be lower, but there are also times when it can spike dramatically, especially if you're popping the lid on long-suppressed feelings.

If you do feel some relief, but you don't feel the issue is completely resolved, a good question to ask yourself is, "What makes this not a 0? What's left?" This question will often reveal a deeper level of subconscious memories or emotions associated with the presenting distress. Whatever occurs, if you're not yet at a 0, go back to step 1 and begin the process all over again. The goal is to get your SUD to a 0.

Let's Do Some Tapping

Wanna give it a try? Here's a warm-up exercise called "The Constricted Breathing Technique" that will help you get used to the process of Tapping.

Begin by taking a breath. (No special breath, just an ordinary breath.) Using the SUD scale, how open or constricted does your breathing feel? (In this exercise, 0 is completely open, and 10 is completely constricted.) When you have your SUD, use the following Tapping guide to help open up your breathing. Please feel free to use your own words instead of the ones written here.

Tapping Guide 2.1: Constricted Breathing Technique

SETUP STATEMENT: *Even though my breathing feels constricted, I deeply love and completely accept myself.* (Say aloud one to three times.)

Top of the head: *This constricted breathing—*

Eyebrow: *My breathing feels tight.*

Side of the eye: *This constricted breathing—*

Under the eye: *I'd love to open up my breathing,*

Under the nose: *But right now it feels constricted.*

Under the mouth: *This constricted breathing—*

Collarbone: *I accept myself where I'm at.*

Under arm: *This constricted breathing—*

(Remeasure your breath. What SUD would you give it now? If your breath still feels tight, do a few more rounds, changing up the words this time.)

SETUP STATEMENT: *Even though my breathing still feels constricted, I deeply love and completely accept myself.* (Say aloud one to three times.)

Top of the head: *My breathing still feels constricted.*

Eyebrow: *It's still a little tight.*

Side of the eye: *I would love to breathe more deeply.*

Under the eye: *It's okay to relax.*

Under the nose: *It's okay to open up my breath.*

Under the mouth: *It's good to take a nice, deep breath.*

Collarbone: *I'm learning how to do this Tapping thing.*

Under arm: *It seems a little weird.*

Top of the head: *My breathing is still a little tight.*

Eyebrow: *I would love for it to open and deepen.*

Side of the eye: *Whether it does or not,*

Under the eye: *I love and accept myself either way.*

Under the nose: *I give my body complete permission to relax.*

Under the mouth: *It's okay now.*

Collarbone: *This constricted breathing—*

Under arm: *It's okay to open up and breathe deeply.*

Take a nice deep breath. How open or tight does your breath feel now? What SUD would you give it? Keep repeating rounds of Tapping until your breathing is as deep as you'd like.

Questions?

What if I can't figure out what to say?

The hardest part of Tapping for most people is trying to figure out what to say, either in the setup statement or in the reminder phrases. There are three things that you can focus on and say aloud when you don't know what to say: (1) the reminder phrase; (2) any emotions that are coming up ("this sadness," "this shame," and so on); and (3) any stressful body sensations you feel (for example, "these butterflies in my stomach" or "this hollow feeling in my chest"). The most important thing to focus on is your emotional state. So if you don't know what to say, just focus on how you feel. If you're highly distressed and just need to cry, then just tap and cry without saying anything.

Do I really have to say, "I deeply love and accept myself"? It feels so hokey!

I understand! The first time I worked with a Tapping practitioner and had to say those words, I became physically nauseated. I thought I was going to throw up. I was shocked to discover that, even after twenty-five years of meditation practice and practicing *kindness toward myself,* the thought of saying "I love myself" made me feel like I was gagging on a hairball. The practitioner I worked with at that time said emphatically, "Say it anyway!" Now, after saying those words both on my own and with my clients and students tens of thousands of times, I can say it and mean it.

In the practice of Tapping, we use the setup statement to relax whatever subconscious resistance we might feel to releasing the stress we're carrying. Self-love and self-acceptance are the antidotes to whatever we're struggling with. If saying, "I deeply love and completely accept myself" feels like too much, try some alternate statements, such as the following. Find the words that work for you:

- "I accept this is where I'm at right now."
- "I give myself kindness and understanding."
- "I love myself as best I can in this moment."
- "I give myself the same compassion I'd give anyone else."

Why focus so much on the negative? Why can't we just do a bunch of affirmations instead?

We focus on the negative in order to clear it. We focus on it because it's there. Even Louise Hay, that *grande dame* of affirmations, once said of Tapping, "You can't clean a house unless you see the dirt!"[1] To put it another way, a wound must be cleaned before a bandage is put on. Unless the subconscious resistance to an affirmation is cleared, the affirmation will be of little use. (I'll talk about this more in chapter 7.)

Does it matter if I tap on all the points? Do I have to tap on them in order?

In short, no and no. EFT is remarkably versatile that way. You can tap on one side or the other, or both simultaneously. Because I often work with clients who carry lots of extra body weight, I often skip the underarm point, because reaching around to that point can be tough. No biggie. Tapping still works.

Can I use Tapping for other issues besides food?

Absolutely! As I mentioned in the previous chapter, try it on everything. And, by the way, even though I just outlined some specific food issues that my clients and students have tapped on with great success, the issue you choose to work on doesn't have to be directly connected to food. If you remember our conversation about stress in the previous chapter, there are many life stresses that can lead us to our food behaviors. Start with whatever is "up" for you.

One final word: while Tapping is a powerful tool for reversing negative beliefs and behavior patterns, it is not a quick-fix panacea. Nor is it a substitute for medical or psychological treatment. Some issues might need lots of Tapping; persistence is essential. If you feel you have emotional issues that require more attention than what the scope of this book can provide, please take responsibility for your health and seek the care of a skilled EFT practitioner or another qualified professional.

Now that you've got the basics of how to tap, in the next chapter we'll begin getting into the "meat and potatoes" issues that can hinder your experience of mindful eating, and I'll guide you in how to use Tapping to address those issues.

For a video introduction on how to tap, visit www.marcellafriel.com/taptasteheal.

PART 2:

Taste

3

You Haven't Failed—
Your Diets Have
Failed You

I've learned to never trust a four-letter word when the first three letters spell "die."

—TARYN BRUMFITT

IT'S FUNNY FOR me to devote a whole chapter of this book to dieting. Because the truth is, I'm in that slim minority of women who have never dieted. Really. Never. Not a single day in my life.

My mother never dieted. My sisters never dieted. Neither did any of my aunts or cousins on the Sicilian side of my family. My matrilineal heritage is of sturdy, stocky, "uneducated" immigrant women who sewed their own clothes and grew their own food and had no time to compare their bodies to fashion models. And other than my sister Patti calling me "thunder thighs" as I rounded the corner toward adolescence, I was never body-shamed inside my family of origin, either.

In my early fifties, however, the combination of perimenopause and a new relationship with a man my body knew I had no business being with conspired to produce a twenty-pound weight gain that formed the dreaded "muffin top" over my jeans. I remember looking at my body with aversive fascination. Whose plump face was this staring back at me in the mirror? I wasn't a full-on fat girl, but when people began asking if I was pregnant, their faces would recoil in an *O* of shock when I replied, "Well, no. But there is this thing that happens around menopause. It's called, uh, weight gain?"

I had enough body-positive awareness to just breathe through it and love myself, but still—I wasn't used to my vulnerability being in such plain sight to the rest of the world. There was no way I could pull my shirt low enough or my sweater tight enough to cover that gut. There was no way to de-puff my puffy face. And I was utterly inept at camouflaging the problem with baggy clothing.

Because I had no prior reference point for being overweight, I likened it to the $22,000 of debt I ran up in my late twenties. Neither condition happened overnight. Both crept into my life like afternoon fog in San Francisco, on "little cat feet," in the words of poet Carl Sandburg[1]—a dollar at a time, a pound at a time, until one day I woke up and thought, "Whoa! How the hell did this happen?" With that shock then came the onerous task of getting out of the undesirable predicament, be it the creditor calls or the visceral flab hanging over my beltline.

In conventional society, the approach to such situations is to *fix* them through some kind of penitential austerity program. Shovel all your money into that infernal hole of debt while you live on cat food. Eat celery sticks and drag your sorry ass to the gym six hours a day.

Which brings me to the topic of dieting. Like budgeting, dieting has its roots in deprivation. The word *budget* comes from the French *bougette*, a tiny drawstring purse you can never carry enough money in. The word *diet* originates in the Greek *diaeta*, one meaning of which was "regimen." Do you get where we're going here?[2]

What's So Bad about Dieting?

It's beyond the scope of this book to talk about money, but I hope you get the idea—or you've already concluded through your own experience—that trying to fix your food and body-weight problems by dieting is, in most cases, an abysmal proposition at best. In the words of Jes Baker,[3] self-proclaimed fat chick and body-positive activist, "[Diets] are mostly unsuccessful, they are usually soul-draining, and they tend to f*ck with your body in negative ways. And they have been something that has caused a lot of emotional and physical suffering my entire life."[4]

Jes is not alone in her experience. Restrictive dieting, in reality, is just a binge waiting to happen. Let's take a look at each of Jes's points in turn.

Diets Are Mostly Unsuccessful

In May 2017, a *TIME* Magazine article tracked the work of Kevin Hall, a scientist at the National Institutes of Health who studied fourteen contestants on *The Biggest Loser* in an attempt to understand the roots of weight-loss success or failure.[5] Of the participants Hall tracked on that television show, some of whom had lost up to a whopping twenty pounds in one week, thirteen of the fourteen regained 66 percent of their original body weight over time.

Hall was stymied to see that, even under seemingly perfect conditions—rigorous workouts, scientifically crafted meal plans, and a team of health professionals at the ready—the bodies of those contestants were determined to get that weight back ASAP.

Research has shown consistently that chronic restrictive dieting is a well-known predictor of weight gain. Dr. Linda Bacon, a researcher and psychotherapist, points out that reduced caloric intake wreaks havoc on the metabolic pathways that would otherwise naturally establish weight stability.[6] The hormonal changes triggered by such upheaval tell your body, "eat less, weigh more."

Hall's and Bacon's observations upend the logic propagated by a $66.3 billion weight-loss industry selling everything from diet pills to meal plans to fancy gym memberships. But in the interest of preserving its hallowed profit margins, that diet industry will never tell you the truth: the more you diet, the more you weigh.

Diets Are Usually Soul-Draining

As a young girl, my client Shelly had no concept of herself as overweight. She was an enthusiastic athlete and a budding actress who enjoyed her body in the unselfconscious manner of a free-spirited prepubescent youngster. But when Shelly was twelve, her mother, who had always obsessed over her own body size, began worrying that Shelly was gaining too much weight and took her to a local diet club meeting.

Shelly vividly recalled "sitting in that hard chair … in a room full of strangers.… I was the youngest there, and they were all so patronizing to me. They were welcoming me into their 'club.' I didn't wanna be in their club. They kept talking about food and diets and points.… When I look back at pictures from that time, I wasn't really a heavy girl. But ever since that meeting, I've felt like I weigh five hundred pounds. Where did that younger, happier me go?"

Shelly's initiation into the weight-watching world cast a pall of shame over her life. She shut herself off from her friends, dropped all her athletic and artistic activities, and dutifully attended weight-loss meetings with her mother. Shelly attributes her decades-long pattern of yo-yo dieting and binge eating, which created two hundred pounds of unwanted body weight, to the misery she felt at those meetings.

As I have witnessed with clients such as Shelly, parents—often mothers—will, with the absolute noblest of intentions, tragically and unconsciously transmit their own body shame to their children and engage their young progeny in a lethal loyalty bond: if I'm gonna diet, you're gonna diet.

According to neurologist Sandra Aamodt, girls who identify themselves as dieters in early adolescence are three times as likely as non-dieters to become overweight within four years.[7] And those preteen dieters are twelve times more likely to develop binge-eating patterns than their non-dieting besties.

When a diet is superimposed over a deep well of self-loathing, it's like shoveling the sidewalk before it stops snowing. By its very nature, dieting engenders the fat-shaming and fat-stigma it's meant to relieve. And the chronic stress of that emotional burden sets loose a chemical swill of stress hormones that keeps the extra weight pinned to your body.

Diets Tend to F*ck with Your Body in Negative Ways

All mammals, when deprived of appropriate caloric intake, will binge eat as a hedge against starvation. For humans with a lifelong pattern of dieting, the brain and body hold the harmful impact of chronic food restriction long after the diet books have been sent to the landfill. In Dr. Bacon's words:[8]

> In the beginning of a diet, you feel a lot of hope, because you are so excited and determined to lose weight, and so you start eating less, and you notice you're losing weight!
>
> Then it gets harder to maintain. Now you're thinking about food all the time, you're conscious of smells, and so on. When your body is calorie deprived, it makes you think about food. It makes sure you don't concentrate on other things, so that you focus on [taking care of yourself by eating]. It even changes your taste perception, so that a wider range of flavors might be interesting to you, so you're more willing to eat anything just to get calories.
>
> But then your body can slow down your metabolism so that you spend a little less energy. So even though you're eating less, your diet is now causing you to gain weight.

Our human body, in its infinite wisdom, is absolutely devoted to self-healing, self-regulation, and survival. One tool our body employs toward that end is *metabolic suppression,* a set point that the body decides is the right weight. This set point differs from person to person—one person's might be one hundred pounds, while another's might be three hundred.

When we engage in calorie-restrictive behaviors, and our body weight drops below that set point, our brain declares a starvation state of emergency and puts a moratorium on all further weight loss until the body is back to "normal." In its mission to get calories into your body no matter what, your brain connives your taste buds into accepting a wider range of flavors. Foods you never would have eaten prior to dieting suddenly become highly appealing. No matter how much willpower you think you have, it's no match for the metabolic smackdown you've set in motion by dieting.

Because I had never dieted, my metabolism is still fairly high, even in my postmenopausal years. For this reason, my body recovered its natural set point once I summoned the courage to leave the relationship while cutting out those oh-so-familiar culprit carbs: bread, pasta, and so on. When I bid farewell to my ex and cut out my bready food choices, the muffin top melted away.

Diets Cause Emotional and Physical Suffering

While writing this chapter, I spent time with a dear old friend, whom I'll call Tina, who spent eleven years in a twelve-step program for food addiction. Three years after leaving the program, in response to life stresses that would bring anyone to their knees, Tina regained the fifty pounds she lost while in food-addiction recovery. Yet, here she was, feeling more grounded, more authentic, and more settled into herself than she had in decades. As Tina confided:

> I'll never go back. Yes, it was helpful for me at the time to weigh and measure my portions and make food plans; and yes, it did help me know what it feels like to be in a skinny body. But even though I worked all twelve steps three times in eleven years, I never got to the roots of my food struggles, which, it turns out, are not at all about the food. For me, the food stuff is connected to much deeper spiritual issues that go back lifetimes, and I couldn't address those core issues while I was obsessed with weighing and measuring.

As of the writing of this book, Tina is still resolving the karmic challenges that have caused her to put the fifty pounds back on, but she's made a conscious decision not to fight her behavior and instead love and accept herself exactly where she's at. She knows that she'll address the food issues when the time feels right.

If you've been a chronic dieter, think for a moment about how much time you have spent obsessing about your food and your body: which diet plan to follow, sticking with it versus going off it, switching from one diet to another, wondering what you'll eat, when you'll eat, how much you *should* eat versus how much you *want* to eat, how much (or how little) you can eat, who you'll be eating with, whether they will think you're a pig if you eat as much as you want to, whether they will love you more if you eat less and are skinny, what you'll eat in public versus what you'll eat alone, how virtuous and pure you feel when you're eating "clean," how shameful and gross you feel when you're bingeing, how you hate your thighs and wish you had that thigh gap you see in all the magazines, how you hate the bat wings under your arms and the way they jiggle when you wave hi to someone, how you can't stand your round belly and can never get it to be washboard-flat like you see in the ads, how your breasts are too small (or too big or too low-hanging or too weird), how your butt is too round or too flat, and on … and on … and on.

Now … take a deep breath … and let me ask you: What might be possible for your life if this obsession were not constantly hijacking your soul? And what do you imagine are the social implications of entire generations of adults—women in particular—being obsessed with and distracted by their body shape and size? What power, creativity, and global transformation might you—and we—give birth to instead?

What's So Bad about Being Fat?

Let's face it: unless you've done some deep inner work or rigorous unlearning, you, like me—like all of us—harbor some not-so-hidden aversion to body fat, whether our own or someone else's. We judge, we crack jokes, and we *"eeew"* someone or something without regard for the impact on those we are shaming.

Unfortunately, we're not alone in this. In 2011, researchers at Arizona State University interviewed seven hundred adults in eight countries—American Samoa, Argentina, Iceland, Mexico, New Zealand, Paraguay, Puerto Rico, and Tanzania—to discover popular beliefs about body weight and body worthiness.[9] Thanks to westernized media images of emaciated supermodels, fat stigma now exists just about everywhere, even in places where zaftig women were once venerated as goddesses of abundance.

Discrimination against large-bodied people is rampant in our society. Patients are less likely to trust the advice of an overweight doctor; large children are more likely to be bullied at school; and overweight women earn, on average, $19,000 less per year than their identically skilled skinny colleagues.[10] Among the myriad misconceptions in our fat-aversive culture is the deeply entrenched belief that overweight and obesity are a one-way ticket to degenerative disease hell and inevitable early death.

After hearing so many of my clients say, "I want to lose weight because I want to be healthy," I began to wonder: Are thinner people *really* healthier and happier than larger people? Is losing weight, in and of itself, the Holy Grail of optimal health and happiness?

It turns out that our culture's view of overweight as uniquely deadly is sorely mistaken. There is no evidence in the world of research that obesity increases mortality.[11] What most studies show is that people considered overweight or mildly to moderately obese live at least as long as, or longer than, people deemed "normal" weight.

Other health factors weigh in as equally if not more dangerous in the battle against morbidity: low fitness levels, smoking, low income levels, and loneliness are all better predictors of early death than a few extra pounds. Overweight people who exercise regularly, don't smoke, and eat lots of fresh fruits and veggies are no more likely to die prematurely than people of "normal" body weight with the same habits. Health improvements in dieters have no relationship to the amount of weight they do or don't lose. And exercise improves health even without weight loss—people who are fat and fit live longer than out-of-shape people with a "normal" body weight.[12]

What Does Work, Then?

Despite how impossible it can be to lose weight by dieting, there are people who have successfully arrived at their desired body weight and been living and loving life in that zone for years. How do they do it?

There's no one-size-fits-all answer. Most people who have sustained their ideal body weight have spent years in a trial-and-error process, trying various approaches until something clicked for them. Some cut carbs. Some cut fat. Some kept detailed track of every meal. Some ate whatever, whenever. Some stopped screen watching and got moving. Some healed their ravaged emotional body. Some restored their body ecology balance. Many use a combination of all of these. What works for your mother or sister or girlfriend or neighbor isn't going to be the same thing that works for you.

In tracking my own clients who have successfully shed unwanted body weight, there is one thing they all have in common: each one went deeper than their desire for weight loss and embarked on an odyssey to uncover, release, and heal the totality of life circumstances that got them into their predicament to begin with. These include repairing the metabolic damages of chronic dieting and restoring hormonal balance; addressing, forgiving, and releasing painful, chronic emotional distress (which is where Tapping comes in); and lowering lifestyle stress by increasing self-care. I'll address all of these in turn in future chapters.

In the case of Shelly, the client I mentioned earlier, her aha moment came when, in revisiting her twelve-year-old experience in that weight-loss meeting, she recognized that she had no power to assert her true will against her mother's desires. When Shelly and I used Tapping to revisit her younger self in that room, she saw this clearly, to her relief and surprise. "I was only twelve years old! I couldn't set boundaries with my mother and so used the body weight both to protect myself and to say no to her. ... I really get it now: my task is to root in self-love so that I can set real boundaries and let go of this weight, which has become a security blanket."

Since then, Shelly's body weight has been in an on-again, off-again fluctuation, with her overall weight progressively diminishing as she learns to love herself more deeply and allow her deeper desires to emerge.

According to Dr. Bacon, "the best way to win the war on fat is to give up the fight." This doesn't mean passive resignation; it means waving a white flag over the relentless obsession with dieting that sucks your life force dry and, instead, investing your precious energy into creating the life you want to live, whatever the number on the scale.

Let's Do Some Tapping

Before we begin Tapping, put this book down for a moment. Place one or both hands on your heart and take three deep, conscious breaths. If you're a frustrated chronic dieter, think back on all those diets you tried, all the exercise regimens you undertook, hoping, "this time it will be for good." Now, contemplate this statement. Say it aloud to yourself. Take it in as deeply as you can:

I have not failed. My diets have failed me.

Close your eyes again and repeat it a few times to yourself, with your hands on your heart. On a percentage scale of 0 to 100, with 100 being absolutely true, how true would you say that statement is? Is it 75 percent true? Or 25 percent true? Find the number that *feels* right to you—not what you *think* is right—and jot it down.

If your percentage is less than 50, and if there's any emotional distress connected to this thought—if you feel shame surfacing, for example—allow that energy to surface. That voice of shame might say, "Of course I've failed! I'm still fat!" Or, "I can't imagine what it would be like to stop blaming myself." Or, "I need to keep blaming myself—otherwise I won't be motivated to make changes." Again, you might want to write these thoughts down. Then tap along with the following Tapping guide.

Tapping Guide 3.1: "I Blame Myself for My Failure"

SETUP STATEMENT: *Even though I blame myself for my failure at dieting, I deeply love and accept myself.* (Say aloud one to three times.)

Top of the head: *It's all my fault.*

Eyebrow: *I feel so ashamed.*

Side of the eye: *Of course I'm a failure.*

Under the eye: *Look at me; I'm still overweight!*

Under the nose: *I'm such a failure.*

Under the mouth: *It's all my fault.*

Collarbone: *I'm lazy and undisciplined.*

Under arm: *It's all my fault that my diets haven't worked.*

Top of the head: *I can't stop blaming myself.*

Eyebrow: *Some part of me needs to keep blaming myself.*

Side of the eye: *Maybe I'm addicted to blaming myself.*

Under the eye: *Maybe it's like a drug I can't give up.*

Under the nose: *I can't stop blaming myself.*

Under the mouth: *I need to keep blaming myself.*

Collarbone: *I need to feel bad about this.*

Under arm: *I'm so attached to blaming myself.*

Top of the head: *But is it true?*

Eyebrow: *Is it really all my fault?*

Side of the eye: *What if diets really don't work?*

Under the eye: *And I've just had the wrong information?*

Under the nose: *Is it really my fault?*

Under the mouth: *What if it weren't my fault?*

Collarbone: *What if there were nothing to be ashamed of?*

Under arm: *What if I could let myself off the hook?*

Top of the head: *I'd love to take a fresh start.*

Eyebrow: *Let all the shame and blame melt away.*

Side of the eye: *Just melt away from my nervous system.*

Under the eye: *All this shame I've been carrying so long.*

Under the nose: *And everything it has meant to me.*

Under the mouth: *I let it all go now.*

Collarbone: *As best I can in this moment,*

Under arm: *I deeply love, accept, and forgive myself.*

Take a nice deep breath. Say the statement aloud to yourself again:

I have not failed. My diets have failed me.

How true does it feel now? What percentage of truth would you give it?

Keep referring to this Tapping guide, substituting your own words where appropriate, until you feel relief.

Tapping Guide 3.2: "I'm Obsessed with Food and Dieting"

If you recognize yourself in those obsessive thoughts I listed earlier in this chapter, use this Tapping guide to help you relax.

SETUP STATEMENT: *Even though I am obsessed with food and dieting, I deeply love and completely accept myself.* (Say aloud one to three times.)

Top of the head: *I'm so obsessed with food and dieting.*

Eyebrow: *It's all I think about.*

Side of the eye: *What should I eat? How much I should eat?*

Under the eye: *Will I gain weight? What will others think?*

Under the nose: *On and on and on.*

Under the mouth: *All this obsessing over food and dieting.*

Collarbone: *I hate that I do this,*

Under arm: *And I have no idea how to stop.*

Top of the head: *This obsession over food and dieting—*

Eyebrow: *It sucks my life force dry.*

Side of the eye: *It doesn't help me get any thinner.*

Under the eye: *It definitely doesn't make me happier.*

Under the nose: *All this obsession—*

Under the mouth: *I wish I could just let it all go.*

Collarbone: *But I have no idea how.*

Under arm: *My whole nervous system is on overload.*

Top of the head: *All this obsession over food and dieting—*

Eyebrow: *How does it help me, anyway?*

Side of the eye: *It just stresses me out.*

Under the eye: *It doesn't help me relax.*

Under the nose: *It doesn't help me think things through.*

Under the mouth: *It just overwhelms my nervous system.*

Collarbone: *It exhausts me.*

Under arm: *And distracts me from what I really want.*

Top of the head: *All this obsession about food and dieting—*

Eyebrow: *What if I could just give it a break?*

Side of the eye: *Let my nervous system know—*

Under the eye: *It's okay to let go of this.*

Under the nose: *I choose right now to release this obsession.*

Under the mouth: *It's safe to let it go.*

Collarbone: *Everything's going to be okay.*

Under arm: *And I deeply love myself exactly as I am in this moment.*

Take a nice deep breath. Check in with your initial distress level—is it higher, lower, or about the same? Keep repeating rounds of Tapping until you feel relief.

In the next chapter I'll help you mine the secret wisdom inside your so-called acts of self-sabotage and see your setbacks through a kinder lens of delayed success.

To tap along with audio recordings of this and other Tapping guides, visit www.marcellafriel.com/taptasteheal.

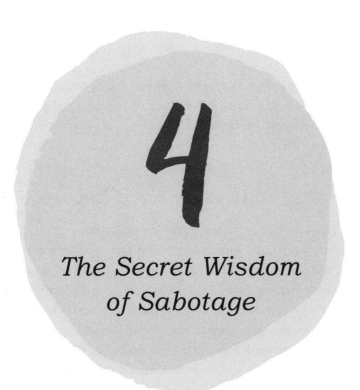

4

The Secret Wisdom of Sabotage

The most fundamental impulse we human beings have is to remain consistent in how we are identified in the eyes of other people.

—STEVE WELLS

WHAT DO YOU feel is the greatest obstacle to your mindful eating practice?

Perhaps you know that you don't crave sugar nearly as much when you start the day with a hearty breakfast, yet you somehow can't muster the motivation to get up a half hour earlier to make it happen. Or you've been diligently tracking your points and calories, then go home one day, bake a chocolate cake, and eat the whole thing yourself. Or you've let go of the white cheddar popcorn, are exercising regularly, and feel great in your body again, but then, when you enthusiastically share your success with your sister, she casually says, "Oh yeah, I tried that too. It never worked for me." Before you know it, you're back in the popcorn, for reasons you can't fathom. Your resolve is lost in the crumbs at the bottom of the bag.

When, despite all your food plans and mindful eating practices, you find yourself still sliding back into old patterns you know you don't want to engage in anymore, something powerful is in the way. Contrary to what you might imagine, it's not God striking you down from Heaven and declaring you a weak-willed fragment of a human who is condemned to snarfing that popcorn for the rest of eternity. However, there's an important issue that you do need to address, and all your efforts to heal your eating habits will come to nil until you do:

Some part of you doesn't want to heal.

Ugh. I know. That probably landed like a punch in the gut. But hear me out.

Uncovering Your False Food Ego

Think for a moment about the things you do well naturally, that you manifest easily in your life and share with your world. Perhaps you are a beautiful singer or a skilled architect or an effortless fundraiser or a whiz-bang database genius. Maybe you have fantastic home-decorating skills, or you know how to make a friend laugh when he's down, or you have a terrific marriage, or you make the best chili on your block, or you're adept at money management.

How is it that you manifest these gifts so easily? You manifest them because they are congruent with your self-identity. They are consistent with how you see yourself and how your world sees you.

Now consider, by contrast, how difficult it's been to stabilize your ideal body weight, or how overwhelmingly hard it has felt to eat three well-balanced meals a day, or how you could never imagine giving up that late-night eating, or how utterly alien it feels to look at yourself in the mirror and genuinely love what you see.

How come? Because these realities are incongruent with your self-identity. They fall outside of the realm of how you think of yourself or how others think of you. They express what I call your *false food ego.*[1]

In traditional Buddhist teachings, the term *ego* refers to the myriad constellations of reference points we employ to tell ourselves and others the story of who we believe we are: my family upbringing, my successes and failures, my education level, my financial status, my capabilities, and so on. If, deep within the recesses of that ego, you harbor karmic residues of old storylines that tell you, subconsciously, "you can't do this," those residues will insidiously spread like weeds and inevitably strangle any attempt you make at progress. In other words, when you are seeking to change your food habits while still identifying yourself with the failures of your past, you don't have enough power in the present to create the future you desire.

The root task, then, lies not in counting points but in reengineering that false food ego at its core to make room for the *you* you want to become. Until you do this, those unresolved residues will keep sucking you back into your old food patterns, convincing you all the while that real healing is impossible.

Belonging Versus Individuating

What causes us to shackle ourselves to that false food ego?

We humans are relational creatures by nature. Despite the radical doctrine of self-sufficiency that permeates modern society, one of our most profound and primordial needs is to belong. We are connected to each other more deeply than we know. (Years ago, when I worked in a department of nineteen women for a small publishing company, we ladies began to notice, as we tracked the production schedules for our book projects, that we could simultaneously track our menstrual cycles, as they curiously began syncing up with each other just by virtue of sharing office space for months and years at a time.)

When our need to belong subconsciously overshadows our equally strong yet seemingly opposing need to realize our authentic selves, we can become stuck in messy unspoken agreements with others in our tribe, which take the form of *vows, contracts,* and *toxic ties.* Let's look at each of these in turn.

Vows

How often have you said or thought to yourself, "I'll never be like my mother" or "I wanna be just like my father"?

In the words of Deepak Chopra, "Every cell in your body hears what you say." Superficially, it might be a passing thought to rebel against your mother or emulate your father. But when thoughts such as these occur over and over, our subconscious mind dutifully registers them with the loyalty of Aladdin's genie: "Your wish is my command." They become vows we don't even know we are taking.

These include *vows of loyalty* ("I will always …") and *vows of rebellion* ("I will never …").[2] Oftentimes we find ourselves thrashing wildly between the two, as my friend Judy illustrates in this example:

> If I didn't eat, my mother would get all pouty, and her mood would completely change. Then my father would feel angry and disrespected, because to him, eating was everything. So I would rebel against them and say, "F*ck you, I'm not eating." Then I would panic, because I didn't want to lose them, of course, and eat everything in sight.
>
> I really get it now, even to this day—when I don't eat to overfull, I'm saying to my parents, "I don't love you."

My client Rochelle is a quiet, intellectually active woman who, when we began working together, felt extremely ambivalent about losing the hundred extra pounds she was carrying. In the depths of her heart, Rochelle longed for intimacy, sexual and romantic connection, and genuine expression of her true beauty. She felt it nearly impossible, however, to experience those things in the body she was occupying at the time.

When Rochelle and I together investigated the roots of her hesitation, we uncovered a vow that she had subconsciously made with her mother, who was also overweight, who neglected her own appearance and continually slandered slim, well-groomed women in front of Rochelle. Rochelle realized that the strongest bond she had forged with her mother was tied to remaining overweight while feeling unattractive and unhappy so that, together, she and Mom could perpetuate their mutual disdain of thinner women.

If your mother or your sister or your partner or your best friend is unhappy in any area of their life, you might have an unconscious vow with yourself not to outshine them and stay stuck, because you imagine that your happiness and success will only increase their misery by contrast.

In Rochelle's case, to claim her inherent attractiveness and her desire for romance was a treasonous betrayal of her mother. After several sessions of Tapping to relieve Rochelle's fear of individuating herself from her mother, we uncovered deeper layers of grief Rochelle felt about "abandoning" her mother, along with guilt for all the ways she felt responsible for her mother's pain.

In subsequent sessions, as we tapped away the grief and guilt, Rochelle found safety in detaching from her mother's misery while finding new areas of mutual interest that they could bond around. She tentatively experimented with attractive clothing and makeup. She took the initiative to engage in fun, flirtatious repartee with men at social events. She joined a gym, hired a trainer, and found deep joy in the feeling of being fit and energized without worrying about the number on the scale.

As of this writing, Rochelle has become friends with a gentleman whose company she enjoys and whom she believes might be a candidate for romance. From a place of respecting her desires, Rochelle has gently released her loyalty vow to her mother and is creating the life she wants to manifest while allowing her body to find its naturally comfortable size.

In Rochelle's words, "I have this new relationship to eating and especially exercise that I know over time will be reflected in my body, and meanwhile I'll keep living in a way that feels nicer, so much calmer, and less like dieting is an emergency."

You might well be striving for more happiness and fulfillment in your life than anyone else in your entire ancestral lineage ever imagined possible. So my question to you is: how happy, fulfilled, and successful can you be and still be a member of your tribe?

Contracts

One day, while in a consultation call with a woman I'll call Alyssa, I got clued in to the reality of contracts when I heard her say, "I'm the middle of three sisters. My older sister is the pretty one, my younger sister is the smart one, and I'm the chubby one."

All relationships are agreements. Within our agreements with others we decide that you'll play this role; I'll play that role. You're the landlord; I'm the tenant. You're the employer; I'm the employee. You're the bossy older sister; I'm the submissive younger sibling. If you have decided subconsciously—or others have decided for you—that within your tribe, you'll be known as "the chubby one" or "the one who's always trying some new thing but never making any real change," you will remain absolutely loyal to that agreement and derail your progress, because to break through and make real change would not be congruent with that identity. Among the roles that we contractually agree to play within our tribe are these:

- the good one
- the bad one
- the provider
- the caregiver
- the peacemaker
- the moneymaker
- the decision maker
- the rebel
- the crazy one
- the sane one
- the one who failed
- the one who succeeded

When Sharyn contacted me to help her overcome her sugar addiction, we discovered a "good girl" contract she had entered into with her alcoholic, low-functioning sister who had been living nearly rent-free in the house Sharyn and her husband owned right next door.

Because Sharyn felt her sister had a harder childhood than she did and because her sister struggled to keep herself and her children afloat financially, Sharyn felt that she simply could not ask her sister to pay the four-hundred-dollar monthly rent they had originally agreed on; nor did Sharyn have the heart to evict her sister and turn her and her two boys out on the street.

In our Tapping work together, Sharyn slowly began to realize the stressful toll that her "good girl" contract was taking on both her nervous system and her marriage, which, in turn, was causing her to reach for the sugar to soothe herself. After several episodes of Tapping, when she was ready, Sharyn summoned the support and strength she needed to ask her sister to leave. The initial confrontation escalated into an ugly, horrible exchange, but Sharyn remained strong and calm. By taking this courageous step, Sharyn traded in her "good girl" contract for a more authentic relationship to herself and her entire family. As a result of that dramatically reduced stress load, Sharyn is having an easier time saying no to the sugar.

Toxic Ties

Relationships that are defined by *toxic ties* are ones in which you have a truth you need to speak to the other person, but you cannot summon the courage to speak directly, and you feel you have no power to change the dynamic. You allow the other person to be in charge of the relationship and then walk on eggshells around them. Because you are intimidated by that person's neurosis, you shape-shift your personality around the unhealthiest parts of who they are.

Kat loved her job and, on most days, enjoyed working with her boss—except during those occasional episodes when he would casually toss out inappropriate sexual comments in her presence. When I asked Kat what stood in the way, emotionally, of her losing the forty pounds she wanted to release from her body, she realized she didn't want to deal with the inevitable sexual attention she would get from him. The extra weight allowed Kat to feel that she was seen as a competent colleague rather than a sexual object. The thought of confronting her boss on his remarks filled her with dread, and she had zero desire to look for work elsewhere.

Kat has chosen, for the time being, to stay in the painful comfort of tolerating her boss's abuses rather than take the uncomfortable risk of addressing the issue. And because she deserves to "treat" herself after a hard day of dealing with him, she continues to stop by an ice cream shop on her way home from work on the days he acts out.

The Secret Wisdom of Sabotage

Let's now come full circle to what I said at the beginning of this chapter: some part of you doesn't want to heal. If you are seeking to heal your mindless eating without addressing the vows, contracts, and toxic ties that are holding you back, your efforts to heal eventually will default to what we commonly think of as *sabotage*—which really isn't sabotage at all.

Why not?

Because your body, your psyche, and your soul, in all their wisdom, are employing those acts of so-called sabotage to ensure that you continue to belong to your tribe, which is, as previously mentioned, one of the most profound needs we have. While we consciously long to change and heal, a deeper, less-conscious part of us would rather stay safe inside our comfortable and perversely satisfying pain than risk the power and visibility that come from allowing our tribe to witness us as having changed.

So when you seemingly thwart your progress, consider that the part of you that needs love, protection, and safety is stepping in at that breakthrough point and saying, "Nope, we're not going any further. We're going back to where we came from." Your acts of self-sabotage, seen in this light, have never, ever been about failure or weakness. They have been your soul's way of slowing down progress when it hasn't felt safe to proceed.

From Judge to Witness

I hope the information in this chapter has already begun to loosen up whatever stranglehold of freakishness you might have been feeling or whatever belief you have carried that you're too damaged to heal. In reality, there's a profound wisdom to every binge, every act of backtracking, every about-face you have ever made in your food journey.

However, despite the inherent wisdom in our sabotage, those actions do become problematic when we have outgrown them and are ready for a different experience. To create the miracle you are seeking in your relationship with your food, you need to have your energy in present time. There is no way to heal while continuing to carry the residual toxins of an unresolved past. What is the path, then, to untangling ourselves from these seemingly intractable vows, contracts, and toxic ties we have with others and within ourselves?

The first step is to arrest the harsh self-judgment you impose on yourself and stop it in its tracks. Judging yourself, punishing yourself, berating yourself will never bring you the freedom you desire. (This is akin to rejecting the absurdity in the statement "the beatings will continue until morale improves.") Tapping is an excellent tool for diffusing the emotional triggers associated with harsh self-judgment, so that you can then begin simply to witness the dynamics of your relationships without them meaning anything further about you.

When the harsh self-judgment has been pacified, you can then dispassionately witness your thoughts, feelings, beliefs, and behaviors and gain the compassion, strength, and power you need to renegotiate your vows, contracts, and toxic ties, for your highest good and the highest good of all concerned. Aladdin's genie is then truly at your command, bringing you all you ever desired and much more.

Let's Do Some Tapping

Begin by placing your hands on your heart, taking three deep, conscious breaths, and bringing yourself into a state of stillness, as best you can. This will allow you to shift into the witness mode I just described. Then contemplate the following questions. You might also want to journal on them:

- Where and to whom have I given away my power? (This might include people and circumstances in your past that still feel unresolved. Be as specific as you can.)

- What subconscious vows have I made? Whom do I have contracts with? Where do my ties with others feel toxic?

- What has been the cost of this loss of power? How is the cost showing up in my food and my body?

🐦 What am I ready to release immediately? What am I not yet ready to release?

🐦 Can I find the place in myself that gives me permission to create new agreements? If not, what's in the way?

Pay attention to any images or memories that float up to the surface from your subconscious, even if they don't make sense. Just roll with it. Of all the stories that are emerging from your inquiry, choose the one that feels the most emotionally charged for you. (In Tapping, there's what's called the *generalization effect:* if you can resolve the most stressful episodes, the smaller ones will often follow.)

Tapping Guide 4.1: Releasing Subconscious Agreements and Reclaiming Your Power in Relationship

SETUP STATEMENT: *Even though I've given away my power with [insert name], I deeply love and accept myself.* (Say aloud one to three times.)

Top of the head: *I've given away my power.*

Eyebrow: *These toxic agreements with [name].*

Side of the eye: *I've subconsciously agreed to [or not to] …*

Under the eye: *And I feel sad and stuck about it.*

Under the nose: *I have no idea how to release this.*

Under the mouth: *Maybe some part of me isn't yet ready.*

Collarbone: *Maybe some part of me needs to stay in it for now.*

Under arm: *I might not be ready yet to release this.*

Top of the head: *But I would love to find a way to release this easily.*

Eyebrow: *Even if I'm not entirely ready to let it go,*

Side of the eye: *Even if I can't imagine how,*

Under the eye: *Even if it might be scary or difficult,*

Under the nose: *I really want to heal this.*

Under the mouth: *I don't want to keep this anymore.*

Collarbone: *I can't imagine letting it go.*

Under arm: *And I choose to let it go anyway.*

Top of the head: *As best I can in this moment,*

Eyebrow: *I release these agreements.*

Side of the eye: *I'm letting go now,*

Under the eye: *As best I can in this moment.*

Under the nose: *I'm releasing these agreements from my system.*

Under the mouth: *I'm releasing these agreements from my cell tissue.*

Collarbone: *It's safe to let it go.*

Under arm: *I'm letting it go now.*

Top of the head: *And I vow, in its place,*

Eyebrow: *To be true to myself as best I can,*

Side of the eye: *Even if that also feels unfamiliar.*

Under the eye: *I choose to be real with everyone I know,*

Under the nose: *To be my honest, authentic self.*

Under the mouth: *I choose this as best I can today,*

Collarbone: *For my own highest good,*

Under arm: *And the highest good of everyone else.*

Take a nice deep breath. Check in with your initial distress level—is it higher, lower, or about the same? Keep repeating rounds of Tapping until you feel relief.

In order to realize the transformation you seek in your life, you must trade in your old identity as someone who *can't* or someone who *fails* for a new identity as someone who *can,* which might mean that you have to step outside of your family identity as well. If that seems like a daunting task, use the following Tapping guide to help you get there.

Tapping Guide 4.2: From Failure to Success

SETUP STATEMENT: *Even though I am so deeply identified with my past failures that I can't imagine ever succeeding, I deeply love and completely accept myself.* (Say aloud one to three times.)

Top of the head: *I have failed so many times.*

Eyebrow: *I can't imagine ever succeeding.*

Side of the eye: *I'm so used to struggling and failing.*

Under the eye: *It just feels like who I am.*

Under the nose: *People like me don't succeed,*

Under the mouth: *Heal my food, lose weight, and keep it off.*

Collarbone: *Maybe other people can do it.*

Under arm: *But I sure can't.*

Top of the head: *I'm so used to failure.*

Eyebrow: *Everyone in my family is so used to failure.*

Side of the eye: *I'm just one of the clan!*

Under the eye: *None of us ever succeed at healing our food,*

Under the nose: *Changing our diets, losing weight.*

Under the mouth: *That's just not who we are.*

Collarbone: *It feels cast in stone,*

Under arm: *Like I'm condemned to struggle forever.*

Top of the head: *But is it true?*

Eyebrow: *Does it have to be this way?*

Side of the eye: *All this failure—*

Under the eye: *What if it's the prelude to success?*

Under the nose: *Who would I be if I succeeded at this?*

Under the mouth: *Could I still belong to my family?*

Collarbone: *Would I still be loved?*

Under arm: *Or would everyone hate me and be jealous?*

Top of the head: *I really don't know.*

Eyebrow: *And even though it's felt like nothing but failure,*

Side of the eye: *I choose, as best I can in this moment,*

Under the eye: *To let the old stories go,*

Under the nose: *And be open to success.*

Under the mouth: *It's safe to be open to succeeding,*

Collarbone: *One day at a time.*

Under arm: *And I deeply love myself exactly as I am in this moment.*

Take a nice deep breath. Check in with your initial distress level—is it higher, lower, or about the same? Keep repeating rounds of Tapping until you feel relief.

If your desire for harmful foods is too strong to resist, it's not your fault. In the next chapter, I'm going to walk you through the physical, emotional, and spiritual aspects of addiction, which will help you lay down the self-blame and gain traction on the path of healing.

To tap along with audio recordings of this and other Tapping guides, visit www.marcellafriel.com/taptasteheal.

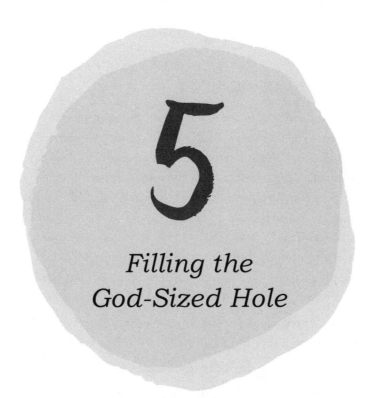

5

Filling the
God-Sized Hole

All addiction is the search for God.

—DEEPAK CHOPRA

IF TOO MUCH is never enough when it comes to your trigger foods, then chances are you're dealing with some form of food addiction. That might be old news to you, as you might readily and casually identify yourself as a sugar or salt addict, or you might chafe against the whole notion of labeling yourself in this way because you associate *addiction* with images of emaciated junkies shooting up in dark alleyways.

Either way, if your desire for harmful foods and behaviors is too strong to resist, and if acting on that desire brings unwanted consequences that create suffering in your life and the lives of others, then you are very likely dealing with an addiction. (I say *very likely* because, ultimately, you're the only one who can decide if you are, in fact, an addict; it's not my or anyone else's job to make that decision for you.)

What does it matter if you're an addict or not? Getting to know your addictive patterns with food will help you understand your food struggles, stop blaming yourself, and begin to turn your circumstances for the better. Let me show you how.

What Is Addiction?

Merriam-Webster defines *addiction* as a "compulsive need for and use of a habit-forming substance (such as heroin, nicotine, or alcohol) characterized by tolerance and well-defined physiological symptoms upon withdrawal; *broadly:* persistent compulsive use of a substance known by the user to be harmful."[1] (If you're wondering what *compulsive* means in this context, here's what *Merriam-Webster* says about *compulsion:* "an irresistible persistent impulse to perform an act [such as excessive hand washing].")[2]

In light of these terms, I want to ask you a few questions right off the bat. We'll use Tapping later in the chapter to address these, but, for now, I invite you to contemplate them, and if you feel so inspired, you could journal on them:

- Does your need for your food or food behaviors feel strong? If so, how strong is it (on a scale of 1 to 10, with 10 being the strongest)?

- Is this substance or behavior irresistible to you? Is your craving persistent?

- Is the food or behavior harmful to you in any way—physically, emotionally, mentally, or spiritually?

- How has your body built a tolerance around the food or the behavior? (For example, you eat more but are less satisfied, or you habitually eat past being full.)

- Do you go into withdrawal when you don't have that food or engage in that behavior? (For example, you might experience headaches, mood swings, or intensified cravings.)

- How does your relationship with food influence your relationships with people? (For example, you avoid certain social events, your partner expresses concern about your food habits, or you choose to eat alone so that no one will see you.)

If these questions are provoking feelings of shame, sadness, and hopelessness, chances are you're struggling with an addiction. If those feelings are so strong that you need to tap right away, go ahead and jump to the end of this chapter. Otherwise, hang in there with me as I unpack the question of addiction a little further.

I'm going to focus on three most common manifestations of addiction, as they are presented in the culture of twelve-step recovery: (1) physical allergy, (2) mental obsession, and (3) spiritual malady. Let's look at each of these in turn.

Physical Allergy

If you beat yourself up around your food struggles and regard yourself as lazy, weak-willed, hopeless, and condemned, I want to suggest that a large part of your struggle is actually outside of the realm of your conscious control. Think about—or, better yet, make a list of—the foods you most struggle with. Let me guess at some of them:

- pastries
- cake
- cookies
- crackers
- bread
- bagels
- muffins
- pasta
- pretzels
- chips
- pizza
- cheese
- ice cream
- pudding
- milk shakes

Then consider this: According to the US Food and Drug Administration, there are over 160 foods that can trigger allergenic reactions,[3] but two of the most highly allergenic foods are wheat and milk products. So if you feel a strong and harmful need to have mini–bear claws or ice cream on a regular basis, you might not only be *addicted* to these foods—you might be *allergic* to them as well and thus be caught in an addiction-allergy cycle whereby your allergic reactions to the foods trigger your craving to have more.[4]

When Julia Child was developing her recipe for a French baguette to be made by American housewives in the 1970s, she wrote that US wheat was much higher in gluten than French wheat, which accounted in part for the difficulty she experienced in achieving the proper "crumb" to the bread.[5] Nowadays, wheat is one of the largest commodity crops in the US industrial agricultural system, keeping dubious company with corn, soybeans, and eggs,[6] each of which is highly allergenic in its own right.

Contrary to popular belief, wheat is not a genetically modified crop, but it has been highly hybridized over the last several decades to maximize yield and increase shelf life. It has also been drenched in chemical fertilizers, pesticides, and herbicides and has been subjected to confounding brave-new-world technologies such as "repetitive cross-back breeding," "chemical sterilization," and "gamma/x-ray seed mutation." So while wheat is not genetically modified per se, it's a genetic alien relative to the ancient varieties that our ancestors ate for millennia.[7]

Moreover, that wheat flour in those mini–bear claws has also been *denatured.* In its natural state, wheat is an abundant and beneficial source of vitamins, minerals, and fiber. When the bran, germ, and other parts of the plant that contain those nutrients are removed, the grain is stripped of its beneficial properties and becomes the bland food-like derivative we've come to call *bread* (which makes me *Wonder*—how they can call it *Bread*). In addition, bleaching and bromating agents are often added to wheat flour, and the nutritional value or safety of these neo-food chemical products is still anybody's guess.[8]

As for dairy products, that processed white liquid in our supermarkets today is a far cry from the fresh, raw product that Farmer Brown milked from his favorite heifer in the days of yore.

As a kid, I remember learning in grade school about the wonders of pasteurization. Louis Pasteur, the nineteenth-century French microbiologist who discovered that sanitizing milk inhibited microbial contamination, was incontrovertibly venerated as the patron saint of modern food safety and singlehandedly credited with making the world a better place for us all. These days, however, milk pasteurization—that is, the practice of heating milk to kill pathogenic bacteria and other malevolent organisms—has come under fire as a devious practice resulting in denatured (i.e., dead) milk devoid of any nutritional value and that produces pro-inflammatory allergenic reactions in the body.[9]

Likewise, the homogenization of milk, in which large globules of milk fat are pressurized and shattered to keep the cream and milk blended,[10] and the defatting of milk, in which the liquid is spun through a centrifuge to spin out the fat, are now believed by many to contribute to lactose (milk sugar) and casein (milk protein) allergic reactions.[11]

Consuming addictive-allergenic food-like products such as these will change your brain chemistry in much the same way that alcohol and drugs do. While ingesting the substances, your brain gets happy-happy-high on dopamine, the neurotransmitter that lights up the reward center of your brain. Processed foods, in particular, cause dopamine levels to soar much higher than steamed broccoli ever will. Eventually, as your dopamine tolerance builds, your brain starts wanting to balance out the rush and so begins shutting down those dopamine receptors, which sends you seeking out ever more drastic ways of getting your food fix. Whereas one scoop of ice cream used to do the trick, now you need an entire half gallon.[12]

When you try to get the monkey off your back and go cold turkey, you become irritable, you feel cheated, you can't sleep, your brain fogs up, and life just feels like a bitch—until you score another hit. So back into the trigger foods you go, all the while blaming yourself for your so-called lack of willpower. Over time, as you become increasingly enslaved to this cycle, your self-esteem goes lower than the floor, and you start to feel profoundly broken, while your life and health fray around the edges.

Mental Obsession

I remember once talking with my sister about a spate of insomnia she was having. When I suggested that maybe—perhaps—she might consider cutting back on the two to three cups of coffee she drank each morning, she practically reached her hand through the phone line to strangle me.

What if I were to ask you a similar question—to let go of one of your trigger foods for, say, thirty days? Or even a week? How would you feel? What thoughts would run through your mind?

If you asked me to give up alcohol for a month, I would just shrug my shoulders, because there's nothing in my physiological, emotional, or spiritual body that craves alcohol. I can count on one hand the number of drinks I have every few months, so if all the alcohol in the world disappeared tomorrow, it would be just another day for me. If you asked me, on the other hand, to give up chocolate for thirty days, I would get a little more territorial, because I still have a harmful urge to eat chocolate, even though it isn't nearly as strong as it used to be. Still, when a piece of chocolate appears before me, I can go through that push-pull sensation, and the thought of letting it go for an entire month gives me a gloomy feeling that life might not be worth living.

Mental obsession, as it relates to addiction, can show up in different forms, all of which accompany the physical allergy aspect I just described. One form of obsession is rationalizing our choices. Are you familiar with any of these?

- "Oh, it's only one."
- "Everybody else is having it."
- "I've been off it for a few months; it's okay for me to have it."
- "I'm gonna treat myself. I deserve a treat!"

Sometimes these rationalizations carry a snarky little twinge of rebellion:

- "Why can't I have it?"
- "I don't care how fat I get."
- "I don't care how bad it is for me."
- "Don't tell me what to do."
- "It's the only thing I do that's nice for myself."

In the literature of Alcoholics Anonymous there's a story of a man named Jim who had been abstinent from alcohol for several months, who one day while traveling stopped into a diner where he had a sandwich and a glass of milk.[13] Then, as Jim described it, "Suddenly the thought crossed my mind that if I were to put an ounce of whiskey in my milk it couldn't hurt me on a full stomach. I ordered a whiskey and poured it into the milk. I vaguely sensed I was not being any too smart, but felt reassured as I was taking the whiskey on a full stomach."

As the story goes, this episode began yet another trip to the drunk-tank for Jim. Despite everything he knew about himself and his alcoholism, he was powerless over what in the twelve-step world is called "the subtle insanity before the first drink"—that flicker of senseless thought that perversely justifies our addictive behavior.

Another form of mental obsession shows up in the codependent union of shame and secrecy and in their tyrant offspring, control. Addiction thrives in isolation like yeast thrives on sugar. The more you isolate, the more shame you feel, and the more you try to manage the addiction with the same addicted brain that got you into your predicament to begin with. So you don't keep your trigger foods in the house; you don't eat them on weekends; you only eat them on weekends; you switch from junk-foody cookies to health-foody cookies; you say you're not going to have more than three; you make promises and pledges all over the place; you commit to a cleanse after the binge; and so on.

But who are you kidding? Such attempts at control usually collapse when presented with the next piece of cake you encounter on an empty stomach. Which spirals you into another round of the shame-secrecy-control cycle.

Another form of mental obsession occurs when we're in abstinence from the food, and then we obsess about avoiding it. This often happens while dieting, which is yet another reason why, in my opinion, diets don't work, because white-knuckling your way through abstinence and mistaking that for healthy food choices means that the trigger food is doing pushups in the corners of your mind, just waiting for the weak link in your chain of resolve to give way. Unless you address the deeper mechanisms of how your brain connives you into these self-soothing and self-harming behaviors to begin with, abstinence, by itself, will never hold up.

Spiritual Malady

All genuine spiritual traditions have teachings about the innate wholeness of human beings. In Buddhism, it's said that all sentient beings possess Buddha nature. In the Judeo-Christian teachings, we say that all beings are born in the image and likeness of God. To the degree that we experience ourselves as separate or alienated from that awakened nature is the degree to which we'll employ our addictions to get back to the garden.

The story of Adam and Eve in the Garden of Eden—which might well be the oldest story of food addiction on record—paints a clear picture of spiritual malady. The story begins with Adam and Eve groovin' in the garden of paradise, naked and unashamed. They're living in a state of *unity*, which in various spiritual traditions is referred to as *primordial purity, atman, non-duality, God consciousness,* and so on. But there's one hitch: to remain in this blissful state, they must never eat the fruit from the Tree of the Knowledge of Good and Evil.

What happens? Eve goes to the tree and encounters a serpent, who says, "You know, Eve—God told you not to eat this fruit, but the reason why he told you that is because he doesn't want you to be like him. He's a paranoid dude. But if you eat the fruit, you'll actually become like God."

Eve likes this idea, so she eats the fruit (which, in various interpretations, is a pear, a fig, a pomegranate, an apricot, a grape, or even a hallucinogenic mushroom[14]), she offers the fruit to Adam, and the next thing they know, they're kicked out. Their blissful primordial unity has shattered into the suffering of duality. They become conscious of their naked bodies and perceive themselves as alienated from themselves, from each other, and from Mother Nature herself.

Now think about what happens when we eat those first few spoonfuls of ice cream, those first few bites of chocolate, that first cookie. How do we describe that experience? Think of all the marketing and advertising terms that are used—"heavenly," "divine," "blissful," "orgasmic." For those precious few moments, our dopamine receptors light up like a pinball machine, and we experience peace, reconnection, and belonging. (Addiction expert Gabor Maté quotes a woman describing her first hit of heroin as a "warm hug.")[15] But as with any addiction, it's only a matter of time until the high subsides, and then we're not just back where we started, we're actually worse off than before, feeling increasingly at odds with ourselves while scheming to recreate the experience.

In twelve-step meeting rooms, you'll hear recovering addicts talk about the *God-sized hole*—a profound, primordial anguish that they seek to alleviate with alcohol, drugs, sex, love, work, money, shopping, porn, cell phones, the internet, fundamentalist religious beliefs, and, of course, food. Where does that God-sized hole come from? As Dr. Maté puts it,

> Neither physiological predispositions nor individual moral failures explain addictions. Chemical and emotional vulnerability are the products of life experience. Childhood memories of serial abandonment or severe physical and psychological abuse are common [among addicts].

> But what of families where there was not abuse, but where parents did their best to provide their children with a secure, nurturing home? One also sees addictions arising in such families. The unseen factor here is the stress the parents themselves lived under, even if they did not recognize it. That stress could come from relationship problems, or from outside circumstances such as economic pressure or political disruption. What we are not aware of in ourselves, we pass on to our children.

> Addicts rarely make the connection between troubled childhood experiences and self-harming habits. They blame themselves—and that is the greatest wound of all, being cut off from their natural self-compassion.

When my own love addiction to the man I referenced in chapter 3 tore my life down to the studs (which I'll tell you more about in the following chapter), I unearthed, using the tool of Tapping, a vivid memory in which that younger me—about eighteen months old—was standing in my crib, crying inconsolably and knowing, in my little-baby heart, that my mother heard me and was choosing not to come.

If my memory is accurate, that personal trauma dovetailed with the assassination of John F. Kennedy, which was perhaps the most profound national trauma of late-twentieth-century America. It also occurred concurrently with my father's going to prison for crimes he committed as a result of the post-traumatic stress disorder he suffered as a veteran of World War II. If Dr. Maté's observation is true, then my mother was no doubt buckling under the weight of these concurrent stresses, not to mention her own addictions, and so left her distraught youngest daughter to fend for herself emotionally.

When we experience ourselves as unloved, wounded, broken, neglected, and unworthy, we are living in exile from our own personal Eden. We then turn to addictions such as food to numb the pain and smooth over the jagged edges of our shattered soul. Curiously, our addictions do just that—not when we indulge in them to the point of oblivion, but rather when we recognize our powerlessness over them, undertake the healing of them as a spiritual path, and use tools such as Tapping to unearth and dispel the traumas and beliefs that caused us to turn to those addictions in the first place.

Addiction is, therefore, in my experience and observation, an intelligent and natural response to traumatic conditions that are bigger than what we can handle at the time. From this point of view, I have come to develop a deep reverence for my own addictions and those of my clients, because, when we heal them at the root, they have the potential to be our most profound journey to spiritual realization and unshakeable inner peace.

Let's Do Some Tapping

If you identify with the scenarios I portrayed in this chapter, please don't blame yourself. It's not your fault. In fact, if all addiction is indeed the search for God, then embedded within the worst of your addictive behaviors is the seed of profound self-discovery and realization. Contemplate the following questions. If you like, you can journal on your answers and then tap along with the Tapping guide that follows.

- What is the nature of my food addiction? You might be addicted to a substance (such as sugar), or you might struggle with a compulsive behavior (such as overeating).

🐾 How does my body feel after I eat this food or act out this behavior? Paying attention to the physical consequences will give you clues as to whether your addiction is also an allergy.

🐾 How do I rationalize or obsess over this behavior? Notice the stories you tell yourself and the behaviors you employ to keep the problem a secret.

🐾 How might my food addiction or compulsion be a spiritual problem? What is the nature of your "God-sized hole," where you feel neglected, abandoned, or unloved? What are your earliest memories of those feelings?

Tapping Guide 5.1: Healing Food Addiction

SETUP STATEMENT: *Even though I'm addicted to this food [or this behavior], I deeply love and forgive myself.* (Say aloud one to three times.)

Top of the head: *I'm completely addicted.*

Eyebrow: *I'm powerless over this addiction.*

Side of the eye: *I feel hopelessly addicted.*

Under the eye: *I can stop for a while, sometimes.*

Under the nose: *Then it's just a matter of time till I act up again.*

Under the mouth: *This addiction—*

Collarbone: *I've tried everything to stop it.*

Under arm: *I can't get it out of my system.*

Top of the head: *I'm totally powerless over it.*

Eyebrow: *Some part of me still wants control.*

Side of the eye: *It's useless.*

Under the eye: *I've tried a million times.*

Under the nose: *Even though I'm powerless over it.*

Under the mouth: *I choose to love myself exactly as I am.*

Collarbone: *Even though it feels overwhelming and hopeless,*

Under arm: *I choose to love myself even with this.*

Top of the head: *Just for today,*

Eyebrow: *Maybe just for this moment,*

Side of the eye: *I choose to step out of these addictive behaviors.*

Under the eye: *As best I can today,*

Under the nose: *I release this addiction from my system.*

Under the mouth: *I clear this addiction from my cell tissue.*

Collarbone: *I clear it from my past and from my future.*

Under arm: *It's safe for me to nourish myself and feel good in my body.*

Top of the head: *I forgive myself completely for this addiction.*

Eyebrow: *My nervous system was wired for this.*

Side of the eye: *I choose to take the best care of myself that I can today,*

Under the eye: *And make the best choices I can make.*

Under the nose: *I choose to release this addiction, just for today.*

Under the mouth: *I choose to surprise myself*

Collarbone: *With how easily I do this,*

Under arm: *And today I love and accept myself, no matter what.*

Take a nice deep breath. Check in with your initial distress level—is it higher, lower, or about the same? Keep repeating rounds of Tapping until you feel relief.

Tapping Guide 5.2: Filling the God-Sized Hole

SETUP STATEMENT: *Even though I have this deep hole in my being that makes me feel unlovable, unworthy, and undeserving, I deeply love and accept myself.* (Say aloud one to three times.)

Top of the head: *This deep hole in my being—*

Eyebrow: *Feeling so unlovable,*

Side of the eye: *So alone and unworthy—*

Under the eye: *These feelings are so old and deep.*

Under the nose: *I've felt this way for so long.*

Under the mouth: *I can't imagine I could ever be free.*

Collarbone: *This deep hole in me—*

Under arm: *That I try to fill with food—*

Top of the head: *It works a little bit, sometimes.*

Eyebrow: *The food comforts me for a while.*

Side of the eye: *It numbs me out.*

Under the eye: *But later I feel even worse.*

Under the nose: *In the long run, the food makes the hole even bigger.*

Under the mouth: *I'm trying not to feel that hole.*

Collarbone: *But it's not working to numb out with food.*

Under arm: *It only causes more pain.*

Top of the head: *I want to stop running away from this.*

Eyebrow: *All these old feelings that I'm unlovable,*

Side of the eye: *Unworthy, undeserving.*

Under the eye: *This old story—*

Under the nose: *What if it weren't true?*

Under the mouth: *What if I'm okay exactly as I am?*

Collarbone: *What if I were lovable and deserving*

Under arm: *And didn't have to reach for the food?*

Top of the head: *This God-sized hole—*

Eyebrow: *It's a spiritual sickness.*

Side of the eye: *I invite a spiritual solution*

Under the eye: *To reveal itself to me when I'm ready to see it.*

Under the nose: *I choose to trust that I'm worthy of love.*

Under the mouth: *I invite the world to show me that truth.*

Collarbone: *At the same time,*

Under arm: *I give myself as much love as I can in this moment.*

Take a nice deep breath. Check in with your initial distress level—is it higher, lower, or about the same? Keep repeating rounds of Tapping until you feel relief.

Speaking of love, in the next chapter I'm going to share with you a God-sized hole of my own that I filled, through Tapping, with unconditional self-love. I'll also share with you my formula for bidding your trigger foods a final farewell.

To tap along with audio recordings of this and other Tapping guides, visit www .marcellafriel.com/taptasteheal.

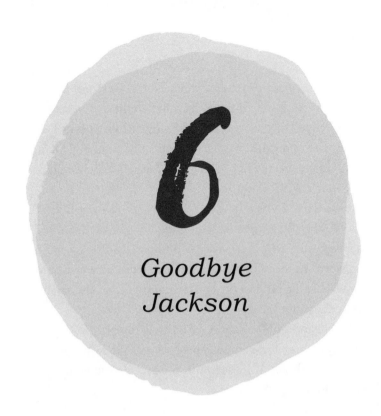

Goodbye Jackson

Pain is the touchstone of all spiritual progress.
—AA TWELVE STEPS AND TWELVE TRADITIONS

BIDDING FAREWELL TO the foods that trigger your mindless eating patterns and freeing yourself from everything they mean to you is more than just getting over your last, worst binge. Breaking up with your trigger foods, once and for all, is about restoring sanity, dignity, and choice to your food behaviors—or cultivating those qualities, if you feel they were never there to begin with.

In the following pages I share with you my roadmap for breaking up with your trigger foods, forged from my own experience and the observations I've garnered from midwifing many of my clients through their journeys. Before I get to that, though, let me share with you a bittersweet story from my own history.

He Was So Handsome

Perfect for me in every way: his lion's mane of thick, wavy chestnut hair; his pale, languid eyes; the angular soccer-player build of his body. I fell head over heels in love with everything about this man (whom I'll call Jackson), right down to his pickup truck with four hundred thousand miles on the original engine.

The life we created together fulfilled so many bucolic visions I had sought to create with the man of my dreams. We spent our days camping, hiking, traveling, meditating outdoors, soaking in hot springs, or delightfully hanging out at home with nothing much to do.

I was in utter bliss. I was also walking perpetually on eggshells. His episodes of aloofness, of not calling when he said he would, of a thousand and one subtle abandonments triggered my deepest, most primordial anxiety. I could never trust that Jackson would be there for me when it mattered. I became a human barnacle of unmet need, clinging for dear life to a relationship that, ultimately, was neither good to me nor good for me.

When Jackson and I hit our nadir, I decisively realized I could no longer stay with him simply because I was afraid of being alone. I knew the gods were playing hardball with me and that, if I was in this much pain, something big was lining up to be healed in my psyche.

"Ok," I conceded to the Universe. "If you want me out of this relationship, take it away from me. I give up."

We parted ways with honorable civility.

In the aftermath of that demise, I made a decision: "I cannot keep attracting this scenario into my life. I can do better. I will learn to love myself enough to say no to that which does not serve my highest good and yes to that which does." I slowly peeled my eyes off Jackson as the cause of my distress and began looking within. This wasn't just the end of my last, worst relationship; this was the culmination of a whole lifetime of neglecting my emotional needs and harming myself in love.

Through Tapping and twelve-step work, I recognized that I had become addicted to Jackson. Now, in withdrawal, I was a love-junkie kicking my drug of choice. I hung on my own personal crucifix for an entire year, crying my way through a box of tissues every single night. Even though I had the support of my amazing Tapping coach, my dear girlfriends, and my abundant arsenal of spiritual tools, I still had to traverse the treacherous terrain of feeling the feelings I had spent a lifetime avoiding and meeting the most brutally wounded parts of my soul.

Eventually I saw, looking at Jackson in my mind's eye, that the physical features of his that I loved so dearly—the hair, eyes, and body build—were uncannily similar to the fantasy mosaic I had pieced together of my phantom father, who went to prison when I was eighteen months old and died there when I was nine. I thought the God-sized hole had been filled: *I had found him at last.* But however benevolent my parting with Jackson, the reawakening of that primal abandonment sparked an anguish that took me to the edges of my sanity.

Over time, leaning on all the supports at my disposal, I slowly flushed the trauma out of my system. Through repeated rounds of Tapping for the little eighteen-month-old me, who couldn't understand why Daddy didn't love her, I came to forgive my father's limited capacity to love because of his own woundedness. His pain never meant anything about my intrinsic goodness as a human being. I was not, and am not, the trauma of my father's behavior. He never meant to hurt *me;* he was just simply hurt.

As the specter of my father's abandonment diminished, I came to recognize myself as deserving of the genuine love I desired, and my relationship with Jackson has since shape-shifted into a friendship marked by a powerful shared history. Unbeknownst to him, Jackson was a medicine man who brought the serpent's venom that almost killed me but instead gave me new life. For that, I am forever grateful.

The Chips Were Just Like Him

The heirloom purple potatoes, the wholesome ingredients, the packaging with its super-hip blue-denim texture, that handsome farmer surveying his pastoral acreage, the hopeful promise that chips fried in coconut oil are nutritionally superior to their highly processed competitors—I adored Jackson's Honest chips just as I adored Jackson the man. And I regularly indulged in them an entire bag at a time—until my stomach felt like it was holding an aircraft carrier.

It was so easy for me to tell myself that this wasn't junk food, really. Come on, purple potatoes and coconut oil! What could possibly be problematic about that? These chips were made just for me. Food guru Michael Pollan says, "Eat all the junk food you want, as long as you make it yourself."[1] Well, if I were making chips at home, I rationalized, they would be just like this. They were my friend, my secret treat, my virtuous indulgence.

As the tummy aches worsened and the charm faded, I had to reconcile myself, reluctantly, to the fact that they, like my ex, were neither good to me nor good for me. Both the man and the chips held out the seductive promise of filling that

God-sized hole for good. They were—and are—*delicious.* But, alas, as the saying goes, "The good is the enemy of the great."

When the time had come to say goodbye to a vision of perfection that, in reality, was only a fantasy, I tapped my way to a breakup with my beloved Jackson's Honest chips using the Tapping exercise I share with you at the end of this chapter. Today, I look at that sexy bag of chips on the health-food store shelf and smile. The chips and my ex alike both remind me that, indeed, with food and with men, I have come to love myself enough to say no to that which does not serve my highest good and yes to that which does.

Breaking Up with Your Trigger Foods

Several months ago, Chanterelle, a student in one of my online classes, had recently received the official diabetes diagnosis from her doc. Among the many processed foods she had to give up in the interest of recovering her health, the hardest was a particular cheese she loved from Trader Joe's.

When Chanterelle and I tapped together to explore her emotional associations with the cheese, we uncovered the grief she felt over having to say goodbye to an old friend who had provided comfort and respite when life's volume got too loud. Chanterelle felt both sadness and relief as she finally understood why letting go had been so hard. Once she cleared the grief with Tapping, Chanterelle found the emotional sobriety she needed to bid her dear old friend a tender farewell.

Making the Decision

We rarely undertake transformational change in our life when things are going well. Transformation usually comes knocking at our door when we're hitting a crisis point: a relationship breakup, a negative health diagnosis, or some other calamitous circumstance. When faced with such situations, we must decide: Am I going to stick my head in the sand, pretend this isn't happening, and hope it goes away? Or will I confront my circumstances, along with all my feelings about those circumstances, and make the changes I need to make, however painful they might be?

The word *decide* literally means "to cut off," or "to resolve at a stroke."[2] When we make a genuine decision, we are not surveying our options as if perusing a clothing catalogue. All middle ground falls away as we recognize: either this changes, or I die.

Embarking on the Journey

In our thirty-days-to-flat-abs culture, we have been mesmerized by the expectation that we should get something for nothing. Pick up a copy of any healthy-lifestyle magazine: everyone's beautiful, everyone's skinny, everyone's doing perfect yoga postures, and everyone's serenely eating their little plates of super-clean birdy food. We are literally being sold an expectation that the path of healing is some kind of spiritual spa treatment.

It's not.

No matter how clear your decision to heal, no matter how effective the resources at your disposal (including Tapping), you are still embarking on a rugged journey in which you will be tested and tempted every step of the way. There are some roadblocks that are common to every healing process—temptation, relapse, and withdrawal—and some universal tools that you can employ to navigate them skillfully.

Temptation

When temptation shows up, as it inevitably does, it's easy to think that something bad or wrong is happening. In reality, temptation is simply the Universe responding to your resolve by asking, with a little wink, "Are you *sure* you want to do this?" Temptation is an archetypal, universal, intrinsic part of every transformational ordeal. All great heroes are tempted: Jesus was tempted by Satan; Buddha was tempted by the Maras; Odysseus was tempted by the Sirens.

Let's imagine that you're with your family at the holiday meal, and you and your sister have been bonded for years around eating the desserts together. You're not doing desserts right now, and she knows it. Yet there she is having a piece of chocolate pie while noticing that you're not, and she gives you a look that says, "Well, are you joining me?" Or perhaps you gobbled down some Starbucks for breakfast, worked your way all through lunch, and are famished by late afternoon. You stop at the supermarket to pick up supper, but your sane decision making has been hijacked by your ravenous hunger, and so you find yourself wanting to load your cart with goodies from the crackers and chips aisle.

When you are tempted, rather than berate yourself, think, "Ah! I'm being tempted. This is a sign of progress." The challenge is not to become discouraged by temptation but rather to become literate in the ways you are vulnerable to it and to resource yourself accordingly.

What are the supports you need to put in place to build your temptation-resistance muscle? In the twelve-step culture, we often use the acronym HALT: don't get too *Hungry*, too *Angry*, too *Lonely*, or too *Tired*. These are what I call "the four pillars of self-care." They are the practices for building a strong foundation of stability not just with your food but also with your entire life.

Don't get too hungry.

When you're trying to curb your cravings or lose weight, it's seductive to think that skipping meals (especially breakfast) is the best and fastest way to slim down and gain control.

Au contraire, ma chère.

As I mentioned in chapter 3, chronic caloric restriction not only sets the stage for weight gain; it also destabilizes your blood-sugar regulation, which keeps you in a heightened state of inflammation and moodiness, which, in turn, totally breaks down your resolve to keep those chocolate-chip cookies at bay.

Stabilizing your blood sugar, then, is the most important hedge you have against junk food cravings and binges, mood swings, and unwanted visceral adipose tissue (a.k.a. gut fat). This means eating the largest and most nutritionally dense meal you can right at the beginning of your day to set yourself up for success, and then making sure you eat full meals throughout the day to keep high-quality, premium fuel in your metabolic tank. This is such an important point that I devote an entire chapter to it later on; for now, just know that balanced blood sugar is the key not only to happy eating but also, indeed, to a happy life.

Don't get too angry.

Like a summer thunderstorm after a sweltering heat wave, the pure energy of anger can clear the air of accumulated pressure. Conflict, handled constructively, can resolve the inevitable resentments that build up in any relationship. Righteous anger, on the other hand—"I'm right, and you're wrong, and how dare you, and I'm gonna give you a piece of my mind and set you straight"—is a one-way ticket on an insane train careening toward a bingeing spree.

So don't get too angry. If you need to blow your gasket, blow it with someone who is not the target of your anger and who can hold the bucket while you disgorge. Tap on the anger and wait until the impulse has subsided before you address your grievance with the offending party.

For many of us, and for women in general, anger is considered a big no-no, so one way our anger can show up is through the Rebel. When you find yourself thinking, "I don't care how fat I get!" "I don't care how bad it is for me!" "I want it, so I'm gonna have it!" then your Rebel is running the show.

Your Rebel, like every other part of your psyche, is trying to love you, protect you, and keep you safe. She might be the part of you that is afraid to fail or, more likely, afraid to succeed. She might, indeed, have some legitimate anger that was never given a safe space to be expressed. She might be afraid of who you will become when you cross over into the vast, unknown territory of healing, and so she wants to keep you "safe" in the familiar pain of your unhealthy food behaviors.

You don't have to reject your Rebel. In fact, just like any unruly child, the more you fight her, the more she will prevail. The key to healing your Rebel is to bring her closer. Listen. See if you can hear what she really needs. Chances are she needs you, the adult, to be the alpha, but she doesn't trust that you're really going to do it, so she hijacks the show. Love and limits together work wonders in bringing the Rebel on board with the positive changes you're seeking to make.

Don't get too lonely.

As I mentioned in the previous chapter, self-harming food behaviors rely on isolation, shame, and secrecy. Our addict brains are dangerous neighborhoods to wander around in all alone.

When we encounter the limits of our abilities to heal our broken relationship with food, we wisely reach out for the support of both a *mentor* who has walked the journey before us and *allies* who walk alongside us and cheer us on. The task of our support system always is to point us in the direction of self-care, self-respect, and self-forgiveness. Where, from that place of loneliness, you might believe there is something deeply wrong with you, your support system only sees things in the way, things that can be moved out of the way as you choose to allow them to be.

Your support system can come to your aid, for example, when you're about to go to the company holiday party, and you know there will be tons of sweets you'll want to eat, or when you're sitting at home at ten at night, and that microwave pizza in the freezer would be awfully good right now. An episode of temptation can be dispelled by a five-minute phone call to a friend who can say, "Yes, I know;

I've been there, too. You got this. You can make a different decision tomorrow, but just for today, don't binge."

Don't get too tired.

If you think your sleep habits have nothing to do with your food choices, think again. When you're too tired, you can't think clearly. Your executive reasoning goes offline, you're more vulnerable to loneliness and negativity, the hormones that store body fat take charge, and, before you know it, that trigger food is in your mouth.

My client Rochelle, whom I mentioned in chapter 4, had a very active Rebel who was in charge of her sleep hygiene. Rochelle's pattern for years had been to crash into bed in the wee hours of the morning without changing out of her day clothes, washing her face, or brushing her teeth. Because she stayed on the computer right up until bedtime, she had a tough time dozing off and often would get right back out of bed and head for the fridge.

When we explored Rochelle's rebellious feelings about her sleep routine, we discovered a college-student logic that thought such renegade sleep habits were "kinda cool" but also "mildly embarrassing." As we tapped on the rebellion and the embarrassment, Rochelle quickly embraced the pleasure of creating a self-nourishing beddie-bye routine that included a fatty snack before bed (to lower her cortisol levels and support deep sleep), along with ablution rituals of her own creation. She reorganized her bedroom to create a less cluttered, more restful, and technologically free space conducive to deep sleep. And she came to attribute the growing peace she made with her body to her new sleep hygiene, along with the increased exercise she was getting at the gym, which also helped her sleep better.

If sleep is a struggle for you, I suggest you create for yourself a "sacred sleep ritual": Turn off electronics an hour (or more) before bedtime and store them somewhere other than your bedroom. Dim the lights in your home. Take a hot bath, do some journaling or light yoga, and say to yourself, aloud, "I'm getting ready for sleep now" or "I'm going to sleep now."

Relapse

The second hurtle to overcome in the process of breaking up with your trigger foods is when you've been "good" for a while, then succumb to some of the twists of logic I mentioned in the previous chapter: "Oh, I'll have just one"; "Everyone else is having one, so I'll have one, too"; "Just one won't hurt"; and so on. Before you know it, "just one" turns into the whole bag, and what follows is a cascade of shame, self-disgust, and bafflement: "How could I?" "What was I thinking?"

Here's what I want to say about relapse: It's kind of necessary. And it can be helpful. This might seem outrageous from the point of view that we're supposed to put down our trigger foods and be done with them once and for all. But here's the problem with that—as I mentioned in the previous chapter, you can become obsessed with eating the food, and you can become obsessed with avoiding the food. The point of genuine healing is to get out of the obsession altogether. From that point of view, relapse, when handled skillfully, presents a tremendous opportunity to forgive yourself, gain valuable self-knowledge, and deepen your commitment to healing.

So if or when you relapse, first, don't beat yourself up. Second, don't beat yourself up. And third … take an inventory of what happened. Use Tapping to tame any negative self-judgment you might be feeling, and then look, with the curiosity of a neutral witness, at the circumstances that preceded the relapse. What was happening? What stress were you under? Where did the "subtle insanity" that rationalized the choice slip in? Were you too hungry, too angry, too lonely, too tired, or some combination of these?

This is where it's especially helpful to have a skillful mentor and sympathetic allies who can review the relapse with you and help you become intimate with and literate in this aspect of your vulnerability. They can help provide you with resources for the next time you find yourself in those circumstances, so you can say, "If I get myself into this situation again, it's just a matter of time until that food is in my mouth, so I need to do it differently this time." Thus relapse strengthens your path and becomes a gateway to freedom.

Withdrawal

Even though I do feel that relapse is an important part of the path, I don't advocate setting out with an intention to relapse. As is said in the twelve-step rooms, "You can't get sober by taking another drink." Clearly, for all the reasons you want to make wiser food choices, there's a need to refrain from eating processed pseudo-foods that don't serve your highest good.

But here's the thing: when you put those foods down, all the feelings you haven't wanted to feel, all of the memories you haven't wanted to remember, all of the emotional residues from relationships that ended badly, all of the unresolved heartaches, and all of the self-doubt and anxiety you've been carrying will surface like a leviathan emerging from the depths of your psyche.

This is *withdrawal:* the physical, emotional, mental, and spiritual upheaval that accompanies the release of any addictive substance or behavior. Physical symptoms of withdrawal can include headaches, nausea, brain fog, fatigue, general malaise, and myriad mysterious aches and pains. Emotionally, we can slip into inexplicable rage, despair, boredom, irritation, and new levels of obsessive fantasy. Mentally, depending on the severity of the withdrawal, we can teeter under the albatross of regret, obsessive self-doubt, and even suicidal ideation. We can become more isolative. Our addictive urges can migrate to other outlets, such as excessive internet or social media surfing, overworking, or codependently trying to control others. We find ourselves jonesing for a hit of something, *anything:* I just want to hear his voice. I just want to have one chip. I just want to be able to eat sugar like a normal person.

I regard withdrawal as *holy hell.* It's hell. There's no way around it. Sugar withdrawal is particularly nefarious, as sugar is well known to be more addictive than cocaine or heroin.[3] However, withdrawal is also holy. It is completely sacred, as it presents an unrivaled opportunity for physical, emotional, and spiritual awakening. I wish I could say this to you as deeply as I know it. Withdrawal is the most rewarding experience you can have in life. Because once you go through, you don't ever have to go back.

The early stages of withdrawal are typically the worst. You might feel exceedingly fragile as you detox physically and emotionally from the foods that used to give you that false sense of comfort. If you undertake the withdrawal consciously, it's important to put in place supports that will help keep you out of HALT: regular meals, adequate sleep, appropriate companionship, spiritual and emotional support, and so on.

As withdrawal progresses, and you move through the pain, especially with the support of Tapping, you gradually feel pieces of your lost soul starting to tiptoe back home to you. You recognize that withdrawal, while painful, is also precious, as it yields to you dividends of restored dignity. As withdrawal subsides, the joy of being alive greets you unbidden. You feel immeasurably grateful for the myriad hidden gifts the journey has given you. You discover a strength and peace you didn't know you were capable of. You not only leave your trigger foods far behind, but you also begin to live the life you have been longing for, anchored in self-love and emotional sobriety. Withdrawal, while hellish indeed, presents you with a unique and unparalleled opportunity to become the whole person you have been wanting to become.

Tapping can alleviate a tremendous amount of the pain associated with withdrawal. To use it successfully, however, I highly recommend that you work with a skilled Tapping practitioner, because withdrawal is not something ever to attempt to go through alone.

Once you become literate in your temptation, make friends with your relapse triggers, and traverse the abyss of withdrawal, you don't have to keep going back to square one whenever you "cheat" or "slip." You no longer have to punish yourself, blame yourself, or tell yourself that healing is impossible. All of the challenges you have ever experienced in your attempts to heal your food shape-shift into powerful allies at your disposal that you can use as fuel to move yourself forward.

Let's Do Some Tapping

I invite you to set before you one of the foods that typically triggers your negative eating habits. If this is a food that you are absolutely out of control with, find something else that's less triggering. You can come back to the red-zone food after you've developed some proficiency with this exercise. It's important, for the purposes of this exercise, that you have some measure of self-restraint, however small.

Set the food before you, place your hands on your heart, and take three deep, conscious breaths. Look closely at your food. Bring all of your attention to it. Pick it up, smell it thoroughly.

Notice the colors, textures, shapes—what are you observing? Take some notes in your journal. If your craving is being activated, how intense is it on a scale of 1 to 10, with 10 being the most intense you can imagine? It's good, for the sake of this exercise, if it's higher than a 5. It might be a bit of torture at first, but bear with me. Put the food down, and begin tapping on the side of your hand.

Tapping Guide 6.1: Breaking Up with Your Trigger Foods

SETUP STATEMENT: *Even though I am intensely craving this food, I deeply and completely love and accept myself.* (Say aloud one to three times.)

Top of the head: *I'm really craving this food.*

Eyebrow: *It's really strong.*

Side of the eye: *I want more than anything to just put it in my mouth.*

Under the eye: *I just want to eat this food.*

Under the nose: *This overwhelming craving—*

Under the mouth: *I wish Marcella would say that I can just eat it already.*

Collarbone: *This intense craving—*

Under arm: *I totally get that this is how I feel.*

Top of the head: *What am I really hungry for, anyway?*

Eyebrow: *What am I really hoping this food will give me?*

Side of the eye: *Maybe it's comfort.*

Under the eye: *Maybe it's reassurance.*

Under the nose: *Maybe it's love.*

Under the mouth: *Maybe it's some feeling that all is well in the world if I have this food.*

Collarbone: *This is a really, really old longing.*

Under arm: *I totally honor it.*

Top of the head: *And I choose to give myself these feelings*

Eyebrow: *Without having to reach for the food,*

Side of the eye: *Because the truth is,*

Under the eye: *This food is good for a little while—*

Under the nose: *A few bites, maybe—*

Under the mouth: *But afterward, I feel pretty bad.*

Collarbone: *I feel pretty gross.*

Under arm: *So this food is not my source.*

Top of the head: *This food's not going to do it for me.*

Eyebrow: *And that's disappointing,*

Side of the eye: *But it's also liberating.*

Under the eye: *I love myself enough to choose what really nourishes me.*

Under the nose: *This intense craving—*

Under the mouth: *It's totally okay for me to feel it.*

Collarbone: *It's totally okay for me to let it go.*

Under arm: *I choose to release this craving now.*

Take a nice deep breath. Check in with your initial distress level—is it higher, lower, or about the same? Keep repeating rounds of Tapping until you feel relief.

Now here comes the moment you've been waiting for—go ahead and eat the food. What's it like now? The point is not that we will never have the food again; the point is to experience the food as it is, without all the emotional turmoil and fight-or-flight baggage that we bring to it.

Tapping Guide 6.2: Making Friends with Your Inner Rebel

SETUP STATEMENT: *Even though I have this Rebel inside me who's in charge of my food choices, I deeply and completely love and accept myself.* (Say aloud one to three times.)

Top of the head: *Oh this Rebel*

Eyebrow: *In charge of my food choices.*

Side of the eye: *I want to eat well.*

Under the eye: *My Rebel says, "Yeah, right—watch this."*

Under the nose: *The Rebel in me binges and overeats.*

Under the mouth: *My Rebel is totally in charge.*

Collarbone: *It's super frustrating.*

Under arm: *I feel like I have no control.*

Top of the head: *All this frustration I feel—*

Eyebrow: *I try hard and succeed for a while,*

Side of the eye: *But then my Rebel comes out,*

Under the eye: *And I binge and overeat.*

Under the nose: *My Rebel takes charge,*

Under the mouth: *And I feel miserable afterward.*

Collarbone: *Such a frustrating, vicious cycle—*

Under arm: *I'd love somehow to let this go.*

Top of the head: *Who is this Rebel, anyway?*

Eyebrow: *What part of me rebels against what I need?*

Side of the eye: *I want to pay attention to this.*

Under the eye: *No judgment, no blame, just attention.*

Under the nose: *I wonder what this rebellion is all about—*

Under the mouth: *All this rebellion.*

Collarbone: *Maybe my Rebel doesn't like success.*

Under arm: *Or maybe my Rebel never got to express anger.*

Top of the head: *I want to tell my Rebel I understand.*

Eyebrow: *Let my Rebel know it's okay.*

Side of the eye: *My Rebel doesn't have to run the show.*

Under the eye: *I'm willing to take charge,*

Under the nose: *Love myself and my Rebel.*

Under the mouth: *My Rebel doesn't have to be in charge anymore.*

Collarbone: *I can lovingly take the wheel from my Rebel,*

Under arm: *So we can both relax and move forward.*

Take a nice deep breath. Check in with your initial distress level—is it higher, lower, or about the same? Keep repeating rounds of Tapping until you feel relief.

In the next chapter I'll give you some surprisingly simple tools for addressing one of the most foundational aspect of any healing process—identifying and releasing negative core beliefs.

To tap along with audio recordings of this and other Tapping guides, visit www .marcellafriel.com/taptasteheal.

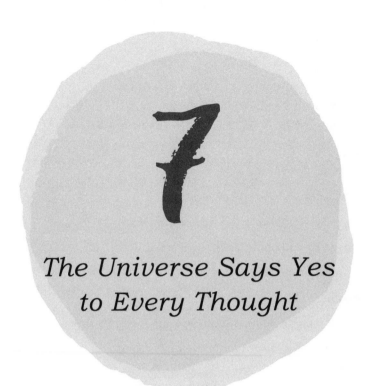

The Universe Says Yes
to Every Thought

Perception is awareness shaped by belief. Beliefs "control" perception. Rewrite beliefs, and you rewrite perception. Rewrite perception, and you rewrite behavior.

—BRUCE LIPTON

WE HAVE NO idea how powerful we are. Every action we take, every word we say, every emotion we feel, and every thought we think create ripples like stones tossed in a pond throughout the forty trillion cells of our body,[1] setting cascades of cause and effect in motion. Whether we are schlepping through the flotsam and jetsam of everyday life or fulfilling our highest spiritual aspirations, creative power courses through us constantly like a mighty cosmic river.

Words, in particular, are perhaps the most powerful creative tools we have at our disposal. Spiritual traditions throughout history have always recognized the word as a catalyst of manifestation. As the Bible states, "In the beginning was the Word, and the Word was made flesh." In Australian Aboriginal society, ancestor-spirits are said to have walked across the earth singing landforms into being. The seemingly gibberish term *abracadabra* is believed to derive from the ancient Aramaic phrase *avra kadavra,* meaning, "I create what I speak."[2] Many scholars believe that the Sanskrit alphabet of ancient India contains analogues for the atoms of creation. Mantras uttered in that language are thought to align our human energies with the vibrations of the universe.[3]

Imagine, then, the cosmic creative power you regularly invoke by thoughts such as these:

- "It's impossible for me to lose weight."
- "I can't control my food cravings."
- "I'm an emotional eater. That's just how it is."
- "I've tried a million diets. I'll never succeed."
- "I'm too damaged to heal."
- "Wanting to be thin means I'm superficial."
- "It's just a matter of time till the weight comes back on."
- "I have to work so hard for just a little progress."
- "If I take care of myself, I'm being selfish."

Thoughts such as these, fortunately, are not facts. They are beliefs that you adopted unconsciously, most likely as a by-product of stressful early life experiences that hurt you. They're not true in themselves, but they become self-fulfilling as you repeat them over and over—and over and over—as if you had a bad case of hiccups. They become so commonplace that you might not recognize them as beliefs. Or maybe you know they're beliefs, but you can't un-believe them.

Liberating yourself from limiting beliefs is the ground, path, and fruition of any transformational journey. Regardless of how savvy you are spiritually, psychologically, metaphysically, astrologically, numerologically, or cosmologically, if you don't heal your negative core beliefs, all other attempts at healing are window dressing, at best.

Conversely, when you undertake the courageous challenge of dismantling your false, negative beliefs, the Universe bestows on you a magic key to creating the life experiences you desire. But this power does not come unbidden. You must choose it and cultivate it, like Luke Skywalker using the Force. Let me show you how.

Where Beliefs Come From

I invite you to look, in your mind's eye, at yourself as a newborn baby passing through your mother's body and into this world.[4] Utterly helpless (as all human babies are), you depended on your adult caregivers to attend to your every need.[5] Having no language, you did your best to signal your distress to the adults around you through facial expressions, gestures, and vocalizations. Sometimes those adults accurately deciphered your signaling and nurtured you properly. Sometimes they couldn't or didn't. In that fragile, prelingual, precognitive state, you made primitive but powerful decisions based on those earliest experiences about how loved you were, how reliable others were, and how safe you felt in your environment.

As you toddled your way through early childhood, you recorded sense perceptions and subjective experiences in the vast ocean of your subconscious mind, while your reasoning capacity lagged behind, trying to play catch-up. As with every other child between the ages of zero and six, you were in what's commonly called a *hypnagogic trance,* or liminal state of consciousness.[6] In that interval, you lived literally in a dream world, with your nascent cognitive capacities blurring the lines between fantasy and reality. If you heard Daddy say, "One day our ship will come in," you would run to the door and wait for that boat to pull into the driveway.

So imagine what happened to my client Lorraine when, as a six-year-old Jewish girl in the 1950s, her mother, in a moment of frustration with Lorraine's behavior at mealtime, snarled scornfully at her, "If you don't act like a lady at the dinner table, your father and I will send you to the Catholic orphanage!"

An event such as this might be considered a *small-T trauma.* It's not a *big-T trauma,* such as rape or combat, but it's nonetheless a highly stressful experience that leaves a lasting dent on a child's impressionable psyche. In Lorraine's case, she grew up loathing herself as unladylike and unlovable, never feeling comfortable in her body, and ever seeking to soothe her hurt with food.

Beliefs and the Freeze Response

When children such as Lorraine face traumatic circumstances at an early age, they don't have the power to fight the adults who are harming them. And because they depend on those adults for survival, it's not in their interest to run away. Having no option of fight or flight, the only option left is to *freeze* inside the stress of the assault, real or imagined. When a child like Lorraine enters a freeze response, several reactions occur simultaneously:

> *She goes into shock.* Something's happening outside of her normal realm of experience, and it's disorienting.

♞ *She feels isolated.* Even though others might be around, when Mom says, "We'll send you to the Catholic orphanage," her subjective experience is that she's all alone.

♞ *She feels helpless.* She's powerless over Mom's behavior and over her own distress. She's at an utter loss for how to soothe herself and rectify the situation.

♞ *Her world is upended.* People and circumstances that she once thought were reliable suddenly become suspect. Her sense of safety with others and in the world is deeply undermined.

Remember—at six years old, little Lorraine does not yet have the cognitive capacity to reason to herself, "Maybe Mom herself was scared of being sent to a Catholic orphanage and is projecting her fear onto me." Her primitive cognition, combined with the self-centeredness inherent in any child, leaves that little girl with no option other than to believe that Mom's behavior means something's wrong with *her.*

Beliefs and "Trauma Capsules"

In order to survive such an overwhelming experience and continue to function in her young world, little Lorraine has to disassociate from the intensity of her pain and relegate the experience to the hinterlands of her psyche. The disassociation solidifies into what neurologist Robert Scaer[7] calls a *trauma capsule,* where the trauma lives in a timeless limbo in our electromagnetic field.[8]

Until the capsule is opened, and the stressful memory is resolved at the subconscious level, the adult Lorraine will find herself saying, "I know I'm not a bad person, but I still feel that old, deep shame as if it all happened just yesterday." According to Dr. Scaer, there are three phenomena that lie entombed within a trauma capsule:

1. *Sense perceptions:* "I remember the look on Mom's face when she said she would send me to the orphanage"; "I remember the smell of the food on the plate"; "I remember how everyone went quiet"; "I remember the knot in my tummy"; "I remember the sound of her voice when she said those words."

2. *Emotions:* "I felt ashamed and abandoned when she said she would send me to the orphanage."

3. *False cognitions:* "I thought Mommy loved me, but now she's gonna send me to an orphanage, so she must not love me anymore"; "I'm unladylike"; "I'm unlovable."

The false cognitions that we develop as the result of our myriad trauma capsules form the matrix that spawns our negative core beliefs. Over time, trauma capsules "leak" when we encounter a stressful experience in adult life, such as a car collision, a job loss, a divorce, and so on. Even if the current-time distress has nothing to do with our historical trauma, it can present an opportunity to clear the old trauma at its root.

Beliefs and Food Choices

How do our beliefs influence our behaviors with food? According to Kim D'Eramo, a physician specializing in mind-body medicine, at any given moment, only 5 percent of our thoughts are conscious.[9] The other 95 percent murmur beneath our conscious cognition like a deep underwater current. The quality of our emotions—what we feel, how we feel, whether we feel—is the direct result of the quality of our thoughts. The body chemicals that orchestrate our thoughts and emotions are the same ones that ripple through our nervous system, our immune system, and our hormonal system, all of which determine how we burn fat, regulate our digestion, absorb and process nourishment, and eliminate waste, releasing that which no longer serves us.

So do beliefs matter? You bet they do. Just as the Word became flesh, so our thoughts—positive, negative, and neutral—create the bodies we inhabit, the lives we lead, and the world we live in. In just a minute I'm going to show you how to use Tapping to heal your core beliefs, but before we do that, I want to delve into another aspect of how beliefs can show up for us.

"Guiding Stars": A Trauma in Reverse

Only three days into her Whole30 reset, my online student Sonia was already in withdrawal from all the pastries she was missing: "I'm not a great cook, but I love to bake. Baked goods are my weakness. And I know exactly where this comes from. My grandmother's house was a peaceful refuge from the chaos of my parents' constant fighting. She always had some wonderful thing she was baking. It was pure heaven to be in Grandma's kitchen with that fresh cobbler and to know that everything was okay in the moment. How am I going to make it through thirty days without a cobbler?"

In Tapping language, an experience such as Sonia's in Grandma's kitchen is known as a *guiding star*[10]—a blissful experience from our past that we continually attempt to recreate in present time, with progressively diminishing (and potentially destructive) returns. A guiding star can drive your food behaviors as relentlessly as any negative trauma can. Getting hooked on a positive event that you never want to end can create a space-time lockdown akin to a trauma capsule. Every time Sonia gathers her ingredients to bake that cobbler, the associative memory of Grandma's all-protective love washes over her again, and, for a while, all is well in the world.

But no matter how meticulously Sonia seeks to recreate Grandma's perfect cobbler—buying the exact same ingredients, putting the same kind of tablecloth on her kitchen table—Sonia's subconscious knows that she'll never replicate that original happiness exactly. But believing, with a child's logic, that the cobbler is the source of her safety, she will bake and eat legions of them in a futile attempt to create that original feeling of peace and protection. In this way, a guiding-star moment of soaring bliss can often usher in a crash of disappointment, regret, and blistering self-recrimination.

The revelation of a guiding star in your own history can bring either an "aha" of relief or an "oh no" of dread, depending on the intensity of your attachment to it. The task of healing a guiding star such as Sonia's is not to take the cobbler away, per se, but to recognize the cobbler as a *messenger* of safety rather than a *source* of safety. The protection and love that Sonia is seeking can be found through myriad channels besides the cobbler. Sonia's task, with the help of a Tapping mentor, is to allow both herself and that little one who's still seeking refuge from Mom and Dad's fighting to open to all those possibilities.

Uncovering Core Beliefs

Core beliefs often express themselves in the language of a small child, anywhere from zero to six years old. Among the most common are:

- "I'm not good enough."
- "I don't deserve it."
- "It's not safe."
- "I can't do it."
- "I can't have it."

Beliefs such as these, when mummified inside trauma capsules, endlessly attract people and circumstances that conform to and reinforce that belief. So if you find yourself wondering "Why do I keep struggling to lose weight?" or "Why do I keep eating this food, even though I know it's not good for me?" or "Why do I keep attracting this kind of person in my life?" chances are the roots of your struggle lie buried within an (as of yet) unopened trauma capsule.

There are many skilled ways to uncover and release negative core beliefs quickly; I offer you here two methods that have proven most successful for my clients and students. Do one; do both; do what works for you.

Core Beliefs Release #1: Inquiry

Give yourself about twenty minutes of uninterrupted time to do this exercise. Have your journal handy.

Begin by placing your hands on your heart and taking three deep, conscious breaths. You can remain here for a few more moments if you like, until you feel that your mind has shifted into a more focused, settled space. Now call to mind a circumstance that you keep finding yourself in despite your best attempts to liberate yourself from it. It might or might not have to do with food. To help you focus on the issue as deeply as you can, contemplate the following eight questions and jot down your answers in your journal:

1. What keeps happening?
2. How do I feel about it?
3. Where do I experience those feelings in my body?
4. What (if anything) does this circumstance or these feelings remind me of in my history?
5. What do I tell myself about why I have this problem?
6. What have I made this problem mean about me?
7. What would be the best possible outcome of this circumstance?
8. What's in the way of that being my reality right now?

Questions 5, 6, and 8, in particular, contain clues as to the beliefs that undergird this situation.

After you've completed your writing, if your emotions feel highly charged, tap along with the Tapping guide that follows.

Core Beliefs Release #2: Release Your "Tail Enders"

Gary Craig, creator of the EFT Tapping technique, developed a brilliant, lightning-quick way to cut to the chase of discovering and releasing core beliefs.[11] This is where Tapping can work its greatest magic. Give yourself about twenty minutes of uninterrupted time to do this exercise.

Take out your journal. Draw a line down the middle to divide the page in half. On the left side, write an affirmation of your choosing (a positive statement that invokes a particular result that you desire). Your affirmation might sound like one of these:

- "I now lose weight quickly and effortlessly."
- "I always make conscious, self-loving food choices."
- "I deeply love my body exactly as it is in this moment."
- "All the weight I need to lose is releasing from my body right now."
- "I eat only the foods that nourish me deeply."
- "I deserve the love and healing I desire."
- "Food is my friend."

In the right-hand column, write what Gary Craig calls your *tail enders*—the first resistant thoughts that come to mind—without censoring. Your tail enders could sound like some of these:

- "Yeah, right!"
- "What a crock!"
- "That's so hokey, I wanna puke."
- "Not me!"
- "No, I can't."
- "Who are you kidding?"
- "Gimme a break!"

Don't judge the thought. Just write the affirmation again in the left-hand column, the countervailing thought in the right-hand column, over and over, until you feel like you've hit the bedrock of a core belief. This belief might be something like one of these:

- "I don't deserve to be happy."
- "People like me can't lose weight."

&• "I can't change my life."

&• "I can't ask for what I need."

&• "I'll never be good enough."

&• "God is punishing me."

&• "It has to be hard, or it's not real."

One of the most effective and magical applications of Tapping is in using it to clear the difficult emotions and stress responses that cause us to form negative beliefs. Even deeply entrenched beliefs can be excavated and cleared, either by oneself or with the help of a skilled Tapping practitioner.

As Kim D'Eramo explains, morphologic brain changes—new neural pathways—are created every time you clear a negative belief and replace it with a positive thought or behavior. Over time, with persistence, as you practice uncovering and tapping away negative beliefs, they'll have no more pull on your soul or power over your life than the worn-out sneakers under your bed.

As a powerful creator of the universe, you can make a conscious decision to reengineer your thoughts and beliefs so that they serve your highest good and the highest good of all around you. As you practice working with your mind in this way, your relationship with food can shape-shift from a perpetual struggle to a practice of deep self-care.

Let's Do Some Tapping

The guided meditation that follows is adapted from the EFT "Matrix Reimprinting" techniques developed by EFT master Karl Dawson.[12] It will help you get to the roots of a stressful or traumatic experience that, until now, you have been unable to release fully.

Review the answers to your questions in Core Beliefs Release #1. If you unearthed an early-life event that's connected to a negative belief that you'd like to release, I invite you to follow this guided meditation, which is a bit of a departure from the regular Tapping that we've been doing so far. This meditation works best if you have a specific memory to work with; if you don't, it's okay to allow your imagination to fill in the gaps. Also, in this meditation, it is absolutely vital that you, as the adult, are emotionally detached from the pain of your younger self, just as you would be if you were a parent soothing your child. If you find yourself becoming overwhelmed by the experience, you can pause the scene, tap on yourself until you feel calmer, and then resume.

- Close your eyes, place your hands on your heart, and take three deep, conscious breaths. Visualize the episode you want to work on as vividly as you can. If there are others in this scenario, freeze them, so they can't move or speak. The only one that's not frozen is the younger you.

- Step into the scene just as you are now and say hello to your younger self. Explain that you are them from the future, and that you've come to help.

- If the little one gives you permission, you can take them by the hand and let them know that they're not alone anymore.

- Take a moment to tune in to how this younger you feels with the adult you there. Surprised? Relieved? Wary? Confused? Let them know that whatever they're feeling is perfectly fine.

- Ask them to describe to you the distress they're experiencing. Listen to their feelings. Ask them what they've made the experience mean about themselves, about other people, and about their world. Give yourself a moment to tune in to them as they describe their pain to you.

- When they've finished describing what they've gone through, ask them if it would be okay to tap with them. You can explain that it's something you've learned that's helped you feel better, and it might help them feel better as well.

- If they don't feel comfortable with you tapping on them, you can suggest that they watch you tap on yourself, and then they can decide if they'd like to try it. They could also mimic you and tap on themselves. However it happens, it's important that the younger you feels safe and comfortable.

- If they're open to you tapping on them, you can simultaneously visualize yourself tapping on the side of their hand while you tap on your own hand in real time.

I've provided a generic Tapping guide below; please use your own words as appropriate.

Tapping Guide 7.1: Healing Your Wounded Younger Self

SETUP STATEMENT: *Even though you're feeling really bad right now, there's nothing wrong with you, there's nothing bad about you, and it's not your fault. I love you, I'm here for you, and it's going to be okay.* (Say aloud one time.)

Top of the head: *I know you feel really bad,*

Eyebrow: *This is hard,*

Side of the eye: *And you're feeling* [name the feeling].

Under the eye: *It feels so bad,*

Under the nose: *And you think that* [name the belief].

Under the mouth: *All this pain,*

Collarbone: *And everything you've made it mean—*

Under arm: *I know you believe this.*

Top of the head: *I know you think it's really true.*

Eyebrow: *It isn't true at all.*

Side of the eye: *There's nothing wrong with you.*

Under the eye: *This isn't your fault.*

Under the nose: *There's nothing bad about you.*

Under the mouth: *The grownups around you—*

Collarbone: *They're not well, sweetheart,*

Under arm: *They're confused.*

Top of the head: *If they could do better, they would.*

Eyebrow: *But they can't.*

Side of the eye: *The truth is:*

Under the eye: *You're a wonderful kid.*

Under the nose: *You're a great little kid.*

Under the mouth: *The truth is:*

Collarbone: *There's nothing wrong with you or bad about you.*

Stop tapping and take a nice deep breath. Check in with that little one. How are they feeling? If they're still feeling distress, ask them to tell you about it; then do more rounds of Tapping, affirming their goodness and worthiness despite whatever they're going through. Keep repeating rounds of Tapping until their distress is resolved.

When their distress is resolved, ask them what would help them feel even better. They can bring in a friend to be with them; they can do what they wish they had done in the original situation; they can go play in the park; or they can get a hug from you. Whatever it is, create that scene where they're getting what they ask for. Check in with them: How are they feeling now?

(If a guiding star shows up—that is to say, if your little one wants a trigger food such as ice cream to feel better—ask them what they're hoping the food will give them. They might say "comfort" or "safety" or "fun." Whatever they say, you can put the food in their hands and then visualize that the essence of that comfort or safety or fun is streaming out from the food and entering their body. Allow it to fill them up from the tips of their toes to the top of their head, so that they don't need to eat the food, and the food can just dissolve and disappear. Your little one is then left with all the good feelings they wanted the food to give them.)

When their happiness feels strong and complete, you can stop tapping. See this new image of your younger self as vividly as you can.

Allow the new, positive image to pour in through the top of your head and swirl through your brain, letting all your neural pathways know that this is the new association you are creating with that old memory. Let the energy of the new image melt and pour through every cell of your body, letting each cell know that the old trauma is now complete, and all is well.

Place your hands on your heart again. Allow the new image to settle into your heart center. Connect vividly with all the colors, sounds, smells, flavors, and sensations of this new experience, along with all the positive feelings you associate with this scenario.

Take a nice, deep breath. On the exhale, let the image burst out of your heart center like rays bursting out of the sun. Imagine those rays extending all the way down into the depths of the earth and out to the farthest reaches of the universe, so that all of creation now knows that this is the new image associated with this memory.

Let yourself remain here as long as you like. When you feel complete, open your eyes. Reflect back on the original memory that was causing you distress. How does it look to you now? If there is any lingering distress, you can clear it with a few more rounds of Tapping; otherwise, enjoy your newfound freedom!

Repeat this technique as needed for any early memory that causes you distress.

Review the "tail enders" you discovered earlier in this chapter. Which of them feels the most provocative emotionally? And how true does that belief feel to you? Is it 100 percent (or 75 percent or 25 percent)? Jot the number down in your journal.

Then use the following Tapping guide to help you dispel that belief. Repeat as many times as necessary until your belief is at 0 percent.

Tapping Guide 7.2: Clearing Your "Tail Enders"

SETUP STATEMENT: *Even though I have this belief that* [state the belief], *I deeply and completely love and accept myself.* (Say aloud one to three times.)

Top of the head: *This belief that …*

Eyebrow: *This strong belief I have, that …*

Side of the eye: *It feels pretty darn true that …*

Under the eye: *It feels so true that …*

Under the nose: *There's a tiny part of me*

Under the mouth: *That suspects it's not true.*

Collarbone: *But it's hard to imagine*

Under arm: *That it's really not true.*

Top of the head: *This belief that …*

Eyebrow: *It's really old.*

Side of the eye: *I've been believing it for a long time.*

Under the eye: *Some part of me knows it's not true.*

Under the nose: *But it still feels really true.*

Under the mouth: *This old belief that …*

Collarbone: *I totally acknowledge it.*

Under arm: *This is what I've believed.*

Top of the head: *What if this belief isn't true?*

Eyebrow: *What if it's not true?*

Side of the eye: *Is it possible?*

Under the eye: *Can I know, 100 percent, that it's true?*

Under the nose: *What if it's just something I decided a long time ago?*

Under the mouth: *What if I could let it go?*

Collarbone: *Who would I be if I didn't believe it anymore?*

Under arm: *I wonder if I could let it go.*

Top of the head: *This old belief that …*

Eyebrow: *What if I let it dry up?*

Side of the eye: *I can keep believing it if I want to—*

Under the eye: *If I feel I need to—*

Under the nose: *But I don't have to.*

Under the mouth: *It's also fine to just let it go.*

Collarbone: *I love myself either way—*

Under arm: *Exactly as I am in this moment.*

Take a nice deep breath. Check in with your initial distress level—is it higher, lower, or about the same? Keep repeating rounds of Tapping until you feel relief.

In part 2 we looked at all the personal reasons why your struggles with food are not your fault. In part 3 we'll pan the camera out to look at all the social factors that contribute to our collective struggles with food and how we can use Tapping to resolve them personally.

To tap along with audio recordings of this and other Tapping guides, visit www.marcellafriel.com/taptasteheal.

PART 3:

Heal

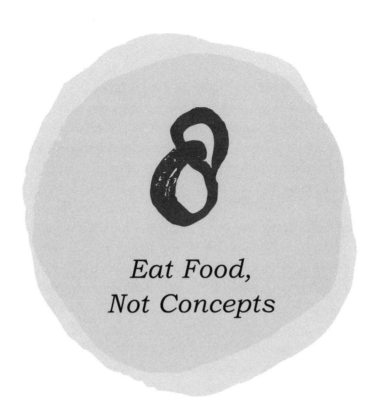

Eat Food,
Not Concepts

*The best and healthiest way to eat is to eat what nature dictates. The challenge
is that we no longer live in a natural world, and navigating that is tricky.*

—SHERRY STRONG

WHEN I WAS a culinary arts student at the Natural Gourmet Institute in New York City, I remember vividly a comment casually tossed out by my beloved mentor, Annemarie Colbin, that landed in my brain like a white-hot ember: "Americans don't eat food. They eat concepts." With her characteristic brilliance, Annemarie summed up our entire food crisis in seven words.

Food culture is the basis of all human culture. Long before supermarkets and food-processing factories, indigenous societies have been (and many still are) anchoring and organizing themselves around the tribal rituals of growing, hunting, harvesting, preparing, and eating food. The reliability of those cycles—planting in the spring, tending in the summer, harvesting in the fall, and storing for the winter—connected human beings directly to each other and to the rhythms of nature. It created a sense of belonging both to the tribe and to the elemental forces that birthed the food on the table.

Just like Mama Bird dropping a worm in Baby Bird's mouth, our female tribal elders—our mothers, aunties, and grandmas—traditionally fed us the foods that their intuition, observation, and direct experience had determined were best. They drew their knowledge from tribal *foodways,* the collective wisdom of a people as it pertains to food: which mushrooms nourish you and which ones kill you; which spices make beans more digestible; why tofu and seaweed combine well for both nutrition and taste. According to Zen chef Edward Espe Brown, those cultures that have preserved traditional foodways have the lowest occurrences of eating disorders.

"Conversely," Brown explains, "we see that ours is a culture with few eating rituals and numerous disorders."[1] In modern industrial society, we've traded in Auntie and Grandma for celebrity chefs, television doctors, nutritionists, apps, recipe blogs, journalists, book authors (ahem), advertisers, food labels, and the latest diet craze.

As a result, we're perpetually confused about what to eat. We judge what's best for us not by listening to our bodies, but by what a celebrity television doctor says; not by how we feel, but by the grams of fat on the nutrition label; not by taste, but by abstractions, such as "60 percent protein, 30 percent carbs, and 10 percent fat."

As Annemarie said, we rely more heavily on concepts than innate wisdom. As a result, we're way too far out of our bodies and way too far up in our heads when it comes to having a clue about what's for dinner. And as so few of us live on the land we came from, we eat a diet that's not only radically different from our ancestral fare; it's a diet that's disembodied from Mother Earth herself.

This is not our fault. A little history might be helpful. Follow me for a moment as I lead you down the rabbit hole of how we got here.

Poisoned Roots

Have you ever had a conversation with someone that sounded like this?

> I was drinking lots of milk to protect my bones against osteoporosis, like the articles I read in the women's magazines recommend. But then I heard that too much milk drinking can actually lead to fractures. "Okay," I said to myself, "then I'll drink soymilk"—because soy is supposed to be good for women. But most soy now is GMO, so forget that. "Alrighty," I thought, "I'll switch to coconut milk." I've been hearing all this cool stuff about how healthy coconut is. But now the American Heart Association says that coconut oil causes heart disease, so I'm not sure...."[2]

This confusion isn't you being dumb. It's the result of the industrial food system's efforts to keep your head continually spinning around what you should eat.

In the years following World War II, the US government funded the conversion of wartime chemicals to civilian agricultural use. Nerve gasses that once killed humans were converted to pesticides; ammonium nitrate, the main chemical used in bomb production, was repurposed as crop fertilizer. Armed with these new products and subsidized by citizen tax dollars, industrial farmers dramatically increased their yields of chemically addicted monocrops such as wheat, corn, and soybeans. With the government picking up the tab, corporate farmers were able to sell the grains for far less than it cost to grow them, which created a surplus that snaked its way up the processed food chain and spawned such dubious techno-foods as high-fructose corn syrup, denatured white flour, and refined soybean oil.

The excess commodity crops also were fed in abundance to cattle, hogs, and other agricultural animals, enabling Americans to eat an unprecedented average of a half-pound of meat per person per day. Thus the industrial farm gave birth to the industrial meat feedlot, with all its social and ecological fallout: groundwater pollution from waste runoff, the devastation of the small family farm and entire farm towns, and the overweight and obesity that cause manifold suffering for nearly 70 percent of the adult population in the United States.[3]

Add the availability of cheap fossil fuels to the mix, and now you know why most people around the United States eat produce from California or Texas rather than nearby farms. The salmon on your dinner plate could be caught in Nova Scotia, shipped to China for processing, then shipped again to the big-box grocery store on the outskirts of your town.

Don't Be Fooled

The justification for this process comes from the food advertising industry, the mouthpiece of the industrial food production system. As no one in their right mind would eat such pseudo-foods if they knew the reality behind the products on their supermarket shelves, advertising provides the systematic and consistent manipulation of the consumer public to keep us betraying our bodies' innate wisdom.

The industry's primary tactic is to deflect consumer attention away from the processed condition of the food and keep it focused on *individual nutrients* as a bulwark of a product's health-supportive properties. Marion Nestle, professor emerita of food studies at New York University, eloquently points out this phenomenon in her landmark book *Food Politics*:[4] "Tropicana, for example, promotes regular orange juice—unfortified—for its content of potassium ('as much as a banana') and Vitamin C ('a full day's supply') and for its natural lack of saturated fats or cholesterol (which are found mainly or only in foods of animal origin)." Nestle then cites Kellogg's Nutri-Grain cereal's health claim that it is "a good source of fiber," about which the cereal adds, "a low-fat diet rich in foods with fiber may reduce the risk of some forms of cancer."

What these promotions hide is that Tropicana orange juice made from concentrate can have a whopping twenty-two grams of sugar (five and a half teaspoons) per serving, and Nutri-Grain bars contain five different kinds of sugar (sugar, dextrose, fructose, corn syrup, and invert sugar), totaling eleven grams (nearly a tablespoon) per serving. The focus on individual nutrients hoodwinks unwitting consumers into believing that what they eat is, in fact, healthy, while concealing the natural nutrients that have been stripped out and the artificial ingredients that have been added, which leave the "food" essentially dead.

Nowhere is the advertising industry's persuasive reach so perniciously demonstrated as in its quest to convert children into lifelong consumers. Eric Schlosser, author of *Fast Food Nation* (in my opinion, the best piece of investigative journalism since Upton Sinclair's *The Jungle*), breaks it down this way: "After largely ignoring children for years, Madison Avenue began [in the 1980s] to scrutinize and pursue them. ... Hoping that nostalgic childhood memories of a brand will lead to a lifetime of purchases, companies now plan 'cradle-to-grave' advertising strategies. They have come to believe [that] ... a person's 'brand loyalty' may begin as early as the age of two. Indeed, market research has found that children often recognize a brand logo before they can recognize their own name."[5]

As children now spend more time screen watching than any other activity in their lives (other than sleep), advertisers can sink their hooks deep into a child's subconscious mind and insidiously build strong brand preferences that influence parents' purchasing choices. Young children (those in the hypnagogic state I referenced in the previous chapter) cannot differentiate advertising messages from program content; nor can they discern the persuasive intent of the ads themselves. Anyone with even an iota of ethics can see, then, that directing these messages at such a vulnerable audience is inherently exploitative.[6]

The Cost of Cultural Rebellion

Industrial culture in general, and US culture in particular, prides itself on *rebellion* against culture. We Americans are a nation of innovators ever desiring to break old molds and make things better.

In doing so, however, we've thrown the baby out with the bath water in destroying the myriad fragile and gorgeous cultural customs that many of our ancestors brought to this land. If, indeed, we are what we eat, we Americans have become a people-less people whose wisdom roots have dissolved in the melting pot, and our distorted food choices reflect our collective alienation.

Divorced from the natural cycles and tribal activity that brought food to us in the past, our industrialized food system erases all context for our food beyond its appearance on the supermarket shelves or in the fast-food menu. That lack of context leaves us prone to food addiction, compulsive overeating, and degenerative disease. The longer the chain between Mother Earth and our food table, the more confused and disembodied our food choices become.

As a granddaughter of Sicilian immigrants who arrived in the United States via Ellis Island, I was blessed to grow up in this country with elders from *il vecchio paese* who imparted on me some of their wisdom foodways. With my father long gone and my mother single-handedly raising five children, my grandparents' home down the street was my day-care center. My grandfather was a consummate gardener, my grandmother an admirable cook. It was at Grandmom Marrone's table that I learned, as early as age four, how to roll pizza dough, grind sausage meat, and pick vegetables from the garden. Because I was continually exposed to fresh, homemade foods, I also developed early on the palate to appreciate distinctive and life-affirming flavors: the piercing bitterness of dandelion, the mild reassurance of zucchini, the deliciously excremental aroma of naturally aged cheeses and cured meats. I learned as a young child the fundaments of feeding myself well and eating good food, so that, even as I wrestled with sugar addiction in my midthirties, I was able to draw on the skill set that was embedded in my gustatory DNA, thanks to Grandmom and Granpop Marrone.

My earliest food memory is of the strawberry patch that bordered the well-manicured lawn of my grandparents' garden. In Grandmom's pink Bakelite bowl I remember staring in anticipatory awe at a cluster of feisty ruby-red strawberries on the verge of spilling their juices. When Grandmom poured in the cream from her pitcher and kissed the bowl with a delicate sprinkle of sugar, I slowly stirred the cream and berries together, watching the red berry ink shamelessly swirl around the dignified cream. My grandfather, seeing my fascination, remarked, "If you keep eating so many berries, the tip of your nose is going to turn into a little strawberry!"

"I wonder how that could happen," I mused, while pondering the red, white, and pink frenzy my delicious treat had become.

As immigrants, my grandparents were always aware of their position as outsiders in mainstream society, and so it was supremely important to them that their children and grandchildren assimilate. Even as we spoke at home in a pidgin Sicilian dialect, they always reminded us that, as *americani,* our survival imperative in the New World was to leave the garden zucchini and dandelion behind and opt instead for the frozen Green Giant *Le Sueur* peas that came from who knows where.

Creating a New Food Culture

While we might feel a poignant nostalgia for the foodways of our ancestors, most of us living in modern society aren't quite ready to chuck it all overboard for a back-to-the-land lifestyle. How do we, then, invoke our ancestral wisdom to guide us in good food choices as we navigate the labyrinth of confusion?

Annemarie Colbin, once again, had the answer. Below are her Seven Criteria for Whole Foods Selection,[7] a fad-proof set of guidelines to help you cut through the endless contradictory information churned out by the industrial food system and crack the code on that ever-vexing question, "What in heaven's name should I eat?"

The criteria that follow are meant to be broad guidelines for how to think about the food on your plate. They are not meant to become something you flagellate yourself with because you ate a salad in the wintertime. Be reasonable. If you apply these criteria to your food choices, you'll find yourself naturally making wiser decisions regardless of whatever food plan you're following.

Seven Criteria of Whole Foods Selection

Whenever possible, choose foods that are

- ⋙ *Whole:* Ideally, all the edible parts of the food are intact: eggs with yolks, chicken with skin and bones, oranges with pulp, rice with bran and germ. Food that has all or most of its edible parts intact has both greater nutritional synergy and more satisfying flavor.

❧ *Natural:* As Mother Nature intended it: as minimally processed as possible. This means staying away from commercially canned, genetically modified, irradiated, artificially colored, and chemically preserved food-like products. When it comes to reading food labels, a good rule of thumb is, "If you can't pronounce it or don't recognize it as food, don't eat it."

❧ *Local:* How "local" is local is up to you. My definition is *not more than a day's drive from where I live.* If my food needs to get on a plane, train, or rig to reach me, it's not my first choice.

❧ *Seasonal:* For most of us in the broad equatorial region of the planet (and climate upheaval notwithstanding), this means sprouts, shoots, and stems in the spring, leaves and fruits in the summer and fall, and roots in the winter. It means eating fresher, less-cooked foods in the warmer months and naturally preserved and slower-cooked foods when it's cooler outside.

❧ *Appropriate:* This has to do with eating in accordance with your constitution. If your forebears hail from the Mediterranean, you are most likely adapted to a broad fare of fresh vegetables and fruits, whole grains, and animal foods in moderation. If your ancestral line traces back to South Asia, you'll want to stick with whole grains and pulses embellished by occasional meats, fresh tropical fruits, and fermented dairy. Those few who hail from the polar regions of the planet, where arable land is scarce, might not have the guts (literally) to digest fibrous plant foods and might be better off sticking primarily to meats and animal fats.

❧ *Balanced:* Look at the food you eat at any given meal. Do the colors on your plate appeal to you visually? Which colors, if any, are missing? Is there a diversity of textures, a balance of raw and cooked, of fermented and fresh? You might not eat a balanced meal one day, but if you seek to balance your overall food intake according to this principle, you will get all the nutrients you need, not to mention the satisfaction of the food itself.

❧ *Delicious:* This is the most important point of all. If it's not delicious, why eat it? Let's be done with that grim "eat-it-it's-good-for-you" ethic from the hippie health-food days. We have lots and lots of ways nowadays to make food both yummy and healthy. And, as all wisdom food traditions know, pleasure is a must when it comes to eating well. So let's make it delicious above all.

Remember: This is about progress, not perfection. The only way to do this 100 percent perfectly is to grow your own vegetables, grains, and fruits in a garden and orchard and raise your own animals for meat and eggs. Beyond that, there will always be some degree of compromise. How much you compromise, though, is up to you.

Out of the Supermarket, into Your Community

One easy (and fun) way to reduce confusion around your food choices is to stop relying on big-box supermarkets as your primary food source and get acquainted with the alternative food supply chains that might well be right under your nose.

This might take some effort—you might have to restructure your schedule or walk a few extra blocks or drive to a town out of your way or get off at the next subway stop—but the myriad dividends you'll receive in return will be more than worth it.

Farmers' Markets

Among the many, many reasons to support local farmers' markets, here are a few of them:

- *Farmers' markets build community.* Strolling around an open-air market brimming with vibrant seasonal foods, you're not only getting easy exercise, but you're also running into folks from town, getting the latest news, and making new friends, some of whom might be the farmers themselves. Back at home, your belly will remember the farmer's smile as he handed you that juicy peach. A bar-scan code just can't give you that kind of love.

- *Farmers' markets support the local economy.* If you stop shopping at the mega grocery store on the outskirts of town, chances are no one would even notice you were gone. If you bring even a fraction of those food dollars to your farmers' market, you're helping farmers keep their farms alive to supply the freshest food money can buy, usually at a reasonable price. Recycling your food dollar in the local economy makes everyone richer. (Hint: If you're short on cash, go to the market a half hour or so before closing. Farmers are often happy to give you extra—for them it's less food they have to reload onto the truck and take home, and for you it stretches your food dollar. Everyone wins, once again.)

    Farmers' markets have higher-quality food. At your local market you'll find a wide variety of fruits, vegetables, and heirloom meats that you cannot find in big stores, because the varieties themselves don't hold up to industrial production. Many foods in farmers' markets were harvested just that morning, as opposed to sitting in refrigerated warehouses for weeks on end, like much of the produce in the big-box stores. Ranchers who raise pastured meats often give their animals happy, healthy lives and are committed to sustainable and humane animal-husbandry practices. And then there's the flavor—ah, the flavor!—you will remember the real tang of a sun-ripened strawberry, the sweetness of summer corn, the tomatoes that make a mess on your cutting board at home, because they can't help but share their juices all over the place. This is what food is supposed to be, people!

Community-Supported Agriculture

Also known as *subscription agriculture,* community-supported agriculture (CSA) differs from farmers' markets in that you purchase a portion of a farm's harvest in advance and then share in both the risk and the reward. The Japanese call this system *teikei,* which means "farming with a face on it."[8] The win-win of a CSA is that you have "food in the bank" for several months, while farmers receive the income they need up front for hiring labor, repairing equipment, purchasing seeds, and so on. Many CSAs also ask that you contribute some volunteer hours to help distribute the food, which nourishes and restores that age-old link of food culture and the human community.

Community Gardening

If you have a green thumb (or would like to cultivate one), community gardening is a great way to build food self-sufficiency while learning new skills (or honing your old ones). Community gardens are an especially powerful vehicle of renewal in urban lower-income neighborhoods, where blighted vacant lots are transformed into patches of paradise, providing abundant health-supportive foods for local residents and raising the quality of living for entire communities.

Smaller Local Markets

When you do have to go to a supermarket, go out of your way to look for the little health-food stores and smaller markets downtown. As with the farmers' markets, CSAs, and community gardens, you'll get to know the folks who work there. The food quality is likely to be fresher and better. The experience is less stressful. And you're keeping your food dollar circulating in the local community economy. For all you know, the owner of that store is a single mom supporting three kids. Wouldn't you rather support her than some corporate big shot in a city far away?

A Final Word

With food, as with everything else, you get what you pay for. If you're thinking to yourself, "Yes, but this food is so expensive," consider this: we here in the United States spend less per capita on our food than any other nation—but we pay the high price of low cost in our soaring rates of degenerative disease.[9]

For decades, the industrial food system has been hell-bent on proliferating obscene amounts of cheap food that makes us sick. Take your power back, vote with your wallet, and rewrite your contract with that system. You will be better off paying the farmer than the doctor.

Let's Do Some Tapping

Still feel confused about what to eat? Use this Tapping guide to dispel the anxiety about making "perfect" food choices.

Tapping Guide 8.1: "I Can't Figure Out What to Eat"

SETUP STATEMENT: *Even though I'm totally confused about what to eat, I deeply and completely love and accept myself.* (Say aloud one to three times.)

Top of the head: *All this confusion I feel.*

Eyebrow: *All this confusion.*

Side of the eye: *I have no idea what to eat.*

Under the eye: *I have no idea whom to listen to.*

Under the nose: *I have no idea how to figure this out.*

Under the mouth: *I feel so confused.*

Collarbone: *I don't know how I'm supposed to eat.*

Under arm: *And it feels really frustrating.*

Top of the head: *I try to be good.*

Eyebrow: *I try to do the right thing.*

Side of the eye: *But I can't figure it out.*

Under the eye: *It's all so confusing.*

Under the nose: *It makes me want to just give up—*

Under the mouth: *And eat whatever.*

Collarbone: *I can't figure it out,*

Under arm: *So why bother?*

Top of the head: *But I want to eat better.*

Eyebrow: *I want to feel better in my body.*

Side of the eye: *I want to stop having so many cravings.*

Under the eye: *I want to feel healthy and well.*

Under the nose: *I'd like to learn how to eat well.*

Under the mouth: *I have no idea if it's possible for me.*

Collarbone: *Maybe it's possible, maybe it's not.*

Under arm: *I have no idea.*

Top of the head: *But maybe it's simpler than I think.*

Eyebrow: *And I don't have to be an expert all at once.*

Side of the eye: *I can try new things and make mistakes.*

Under the eye: *I can learn as I go what feels good to me.*

Under the nose: *It's okay to feel all this confusion.*

Under the mouth: *It's okay to let go of all this confusion.*

Collarbone: *I choose to let it go now.*

Under arm: *And love myself exactly as I am in this moment.*

Take a nice deep breath. Check in with your initial distress level—is it higher, lower, or about the same? Keep repeating rounds of Tapping until you feel relief.

This Tapping guide is for you if you feel confident and knowledgeable about the foods you should be eating, but you still keep lapsing back to the processed stuff anyway.

Tapping Guide 8.2: "I Know What to Eat; I Just Don't Eat It"

SETUP STATEMENT: *Even though I know what I should be eating, but I just don't do it, I deeply love and completely accept myself.* (Say aloud one to three times.)

Top of the head: *I know what to eat.*

Eyebrow: *I have no confusion about that at all.*

Side of the eye: *But I just don't do it.*

Under the eye: *I make food choices that I know are bad for me,*

Under the nose: *And I do it anyway.*

Under the mouth: *It feels baffling and frustrating.*

Collarbone: *I don't get why I do this—*

Under arm: *Despite what I know.*

Top of the head: *I'm still putting junk in my body.*

Eyebrow: *I wish I could stop.*

Side of the eye: *I don't get why I do this.*

Under the eye: *I know better!*

Under the nose: *And here I am stuffing junk in my face.*

Under the mouth: *I feel so frustrated with myself.*

Collarbone: *I would love to make the food choices*

Under arm: *That I know would help me be healthy.*

Top of the head: *But part of me rebels against that.*

Eyebrow: *It's easier to just eat junk.*

Side of the eye: *Healthy food is boring.*

Under the eye: *It's easier to grab some junk food*

Under the nose: *Than it is to eat healthy.*

Under the mouth: *At least that's what I tell myself.*

Collarbone: *That's my story.*

Under arm: *I'm willing to change it.*

Top of the head: *This is an old deep habit.*

Eyebrow: *I'm not sure I can let it go yet.*

Side of the eye: *I totally own that,*

Under the eye: *But I'm willing to be open.*

Under the nose: *Maybe, just maybe,*

Under the mouth: *I could shift someday to eating better.*

Collarbone: *I'm willing to open to it,*

Under arm: *And I appreciate myself for that.*

Take a nice deep breath. Check in with your initial distress level—is it higher, lower, or about the same? Keep repeating rounds of Tapping until you feel relief.

In the following chapter you will learn the most important habit you can develop to tame your food cravings, de-stress your body, and start every day on an even keel.

To tap along with audio recordings of this and other Tapping guides, visit www .marcellafriel.com/taptasteheal.

9

Breakfast: The Key to a Happy Life

Breakfast like a queen; lunch like a princess; supper like a pauper.

—POPULAR SAYING

THOUGH MY MOTHER'S parenting skills weren't the best, she did always make sure I had breakfast in my little belly every morning. Her smoothie was one of my favorites: whole milk, vanilla extract, raw egg (no salmonella in those days), and frozen overripe bananas whirred in the blender. I drank this down, wiped away my milk moustache, and held out my empty glass for more.

During my therapeutic chef training, while reading about the virtues of breakfast, I jumped up from my studies one day to call my mother and thank her for feeding me breakfast all those years. Choking back tears, all she could say was, "You're so welcome, little pumpkin." Thanks to Mom's early training, it's rare for me to start my day on an empty stomach.

The Breakfast–Blood Sugar Connection

You've no doubt heard that breakfast is the most important meal of the day, but do you know *why?* During sleep we abstain from food and drink (unless we're raiding the fridge at three in the morning, but that's another story), so breakfast is, literally, breaking the fast.

Breakfast sets up our blood-sugar balance (or imbalance) for the rest of the day. A breakfast rich in high-quality protein, health-supportive fats, and unrefined complex carbohydrates keeps our blood sugar stable, even if we don't eat a great lunch or supper. Conversely, if we skip breakfast—or snarf down coffee and pastries—our blood sugar spikes, crashes, and never rebalances, even if we eat well the rest of the day.

You might be wondering why you should care about something as seemingly abstract as blood sugar. Thinking about your blood sugar might not feel as compelling as thinking about that muffin top that you'd like to get rid of. But the way to lose the muffin top is through the blood sugar.

How so?

Balanced blood sugar supports balanced hormones, which support balanced body weight. When we suffer from *dysglycemia* (unstable blood sugar), we can gain weight without eating a thing. We're cranky, snarly, weepy, and more prone to stress, which destabilizes our blood sugar further and sets a vicious cycle in motion. Let's take a deeper look at how those mysterious things we call our *hormones* can set us up for success not just in our food sanity and weight-loss efforts but, indeed, in our entire life.

Say Hello to Your Hormones

When your mood is fluctuating wildly, do you often say, to yourself or others, "I'm feeling hormonal"?[1] By this, do you mean, "Invisible forces beyond my control are taking over my mind, like aliens from outer space"?

We've all been there. But here's the thing: your lifestyle choices—your habits, beliefs, and behaviors—all influence your body's hormonal activity and, in turn, are influenced by them. When you really get this, you don't need to blame your bad mood on your PMS or your hot flashes anymore. You don't need to blame anyone (including yourself) for anything, in fact. You just need a little information and support to help you learn which habits keep your hormones happy and which ones send them spiraling. So what are hormones, anyway? And what does "feeling hormonal" really mean?

Hormones are chemical messengers that are created in the glandular system of our body (the hypothalamus, pituitary, thyroid, adrenals, ovaries, testes, and so on). Hormones regulate most major and minor bodily functions, from taking a pee to making a baby. They also govern brain functions that regulate both cognition and mood. There are many hormones—new ones being discovered all the time—but for the purposes of talking about breakfast and food cravings and body weight, I'm going to focus on the three biggies you most need to know about: cortisol, insulin, and leptin.

Cortisol

Cortisol is a hormone released from the body's adrenal glands in response to stress. You probably know cortisol as the hormone that's helpful in an emergency, along with adrenaline. When you need to run out of a burning building or keep somebody's fists from landing on your face, cortisol is your friend. Unlike adrenaline, which binds to receptors on your heart and increases heart rate and respiration, cortisol binds to receptors on your fat cells, liver, and pancreas and tells your body to release stored glucose, which gives you the sharp blood-sugar spike and surge of energy you need to fend off the attack or make a quick exit.

But let's say the "attack" is coming from a really disturbing post on social media (which you're looking at too late at night, when your inner guidance is saying you need to go to sleep). Your cortisol doesn't know the difference between a real-time threat and a screen image, so it dutifully does its job of jolting your energy—but in this case, as you lie there scrolling away, your body has to deal with all that extra glucose in your blood that's not being used in an actual fight-or-flight scenario.

Where does that blood glucose go? If your life is full of myriad, chronic stresses—a nasty boss at work, a daily traffic jam—that excess glucose in your bloodstream can translate directly into *visceral adipose tissue* (gut fat), along with weakened immunological and emotional resilience, which, in turn, makes you crave your trigger foods for relief. In other words, unstable blood sugar makes you vulnerable to weight gain, food cravings, and ever-higher levels of stress.

Ideally, our cortisol levels run higher in the morning, when we need to get up and at 'em, and lower in the evening, when we need to wind down. So one simple way to gauge if your cortisol might be out of whack is to take a look at your energy as you move through the day. Are you hitting the snooze button ten times before getting up? Do you wake up feeling exhausted? And then, at the other end of the day, are you rebelling against getting to bed at a reasonable hour? Do you get a "second wind" that keeps you up into the wee hours, when you'd really like to be sound asleep?[2]

Because cortisol is higher in the morning, an excellent way to nourish your cortisol-producing adrenals is with a hearty breakfast of high-quality protein, health-supportive fats, and unrefined complex carbohydrates. Your cortisol can then do its job of getting you going in the morning, and then it can clock off when nighttime comes around, allowing the relaxation hormones to do their job in helping you sleep like a baby.

Insulin

With all the talk of type 2 diabetes these days, you've no doubt heard of insulin, but you might not know exactly what it is or what it does. Unlike cortisol, which is produced in the adrenal glands, insulin comes from the pancreas and is responsible for keeping blood-sugar (blood glucose) levels on an even keel.

Insulin's job is to escort excess glucose from the blood-stream into cell tissues, where it can be converted into energy. When we eat a high-fiber complex carbohydrate, such as brown rice or black beans, our digestion as a whole is busy converting the complex fibers and starches into energy, so it takes more time for the glucose to enter the bloodstream, which means the insulin can kick back while the rest of the digestion process does its thing.

When we eat a bag of cookies, by contrast, we dump a shite-ton of sugar into our system, without the health-supportive fats, fibers, and proteins that slow down the glycemic uptake. Insulin responds to this assault by flooding the bloodstream to get that crisis handled as quickly as possible. What happens, then, when cookies and such become our everyday fare? How does our body handle a chronic onslaught of refined-carb sugary foods?

As the repeated assault becomes "normal," and insulin keeps working its tail off to get that sugar out of our blood and into our cells, there comes a time our cells shut off their insulin receptors and say to insulin, "no more," leaving the bloodstream to fend for itself. Like a landfill overwhelmed with trash, sugary blood becomes sluggish, thick, and viscous, and it can't flow to all the parts of the body that need nourishment. Our toes, feet, and lower legs pay the price, as do our eyes, with their networks of tiny capillaries that the thick blood can't reach. This is what's called *insulin resistance,* the canary in the coal mine of type 2 diabetes, and it explains why many with this condition tragically lose their lower limbs and eyesight.

Left on its own, with nowhere to go, insulin, ever loyal in its duties, decides that, if the cells won't take the glucose any more, the only option left is to send it to the liver. The liver—a miraculous workhorse of an organ that deserves much more praise than it ever gets—doesn't quite know what to do with it either, so it shores up the glucose up for a rainy day by converting it into *adipose* (fatty) tissue stored around the *viscera* (the internal organs of the body). Hence the condition that many experts describe as *diabesity*—the dual affliction of type 2 diabetes and obesity.

If all that information just left your eyes glazing over, let's look at this insulin issue another way. Imagine that your stomach is a wood stove, your food is the fuel in your stove, and insulin is the fire that consumes the fuel. Eating sugary foods for breakfast, or skipping breakfast altogether, is like throwing paper in a wood stove. It's like being wildly infatuated with someone and thinking that it's true love when you've barely gotten to know them. The paper flares up and burns out in a dramatic flame that leaves nothing in its wake but ashes and misery.

Stabilizing your blood-sugar levels, starting with a good breakfast and having complete meals at regular intervals, is like throwing a well-seasoned log into the stove. It's definitely not as exciting—it might take you a while to chew that high-fiber food or get to know that person you didn't initially notice in the crowded room. It might take a while for the log to ignite—but it gives you a slow, steady, and infinitely more gratifying burn in the longer term. When the log burns down, it leaves coals and embers (minerals and nutrients) that can stoke up a new log in no time. All the high-quality calories you put in your body pay homage to this noble fire and surrender themselves in its service, which means your body burns fat and utilizes nutrients more efficiently. In short, the more steadily you kindle your digestive (and romantic) fire, the better both will function, and the happier you are over the longer term.

Leptin

I want to begin the conversation about leptin by asking you a really strange question: Have you ever wondered how your brain knows whether your body is fat or thin?

If not, let me introduce you to leptin. Discovered in 1994, leptin is now regarded as the master hormone that regulates body weight, activates fat burning, and modulates the palate's appetite for sweets. Leptin also activates the brain's *satiety cues*—it tells the brain when the belly is full.

Leptin is produced directly in fat cells. Its function is to travel through the bloodstream and report to the hypothalamus, the conductor of the glandular orchestra, how much fat you have in your body. When leptin levels are optimal, and its cell receptors are open, you lose your sweet cravings, you fill up quickly on just a few bites, your metabolism speeds up, and you burn fat like a top contestant on *The Biggest Loser*.

Sounds like heaven, right?

Here's the hitch: if you're carrying excess weight that's been hard to lose, whether fifteen pounds or fifty, chances are your hypothalamus has stopped listening to leptin, which is the same as having no leptin at all. You probably know what *leptin resistance* feels like: you eat and eat until you're stuffed, you struggle to lose weight, you crave sweets, and your metabolism slogs along. The more excess weight you carry, the higher your leptin resistance. Just as with insulin resistance (which is triggered by leptin resistance), leptin knocks at the receptors of the brain begging to be let in, but the brain, like a weary spouse who's heard it all before, just tunes it out.

According to weight-loss guru Jon Gabriel,[3] who lost a staggering 220 pounds without dieting, surgery, or punitive exercise in 2004 and has kept it off ever since, leptin resistance is the principal reason you keep gaining back the weight you lost. The biggest activator of leptin resistance is the constellation of conditions he calls the *chronic stress response network*. What makes up that network? You know—the usual suspects:

- poor food choices
- environmental toxins
- chronic isolation and loneliness
- unresolved emotional issues
- financial stress
- lack of sleep and exercise
- lack of play and leisure
- existential anxiety

Chronic stress acts like a dimmer switch that dials down leptin receptors and creates that metabolic set point I mentioned in chapter 3. When your body weight goes below the set point, your hypothalamus says "no way" to leptin's fat-burning agenda and does everything it can to get your back to "normal."

The good news is that leptin resistance can be reversed. Eating a hearty breakfast rich in high-quality fats, protein, and complex carbohydrates is like sending leptin and your brain to marital counseling. They finally have the medium by which they can reopen communications and get your body releasing that extra weight once and for all. A good breakfast eaten regularly increases leptin uptake and lowers the body's metabolic set point, so that those extra pounds can bid the body a final farewell.

What's for Breakfast?

So what is a nourishing breakfast, you might ask? Three nutrients are needed at breakfast to keep your blood sugar on an even keel throughout the day. The first one you probably won't believe.

Fat

If you have been following mainstream dietary advice for the past sixty years, you might well believe, with evangelistic fervor, that fat in food equals fat on your body. If so, you've probably shunned that nine-calorie-per-gram menace like the plague.

I'm so sorry to be the one to break the news to you—and I really wish it weren't true—but, dear reader, you have been deliberately misled to believe this, at great cost to your health and the health of society as a whole.[4] Contrary to everything the food industry has brainwashed you into believing, high-quality fat from whole-food sources is one of your best friends when it comes to curbing unmindful food habits and releasing excess weight. Fat is the food of your brain, and your brain is the sovereign of your belly. When your brain and your belly are in sync, you know, with infinitely greater clarity, when you're hungry, when you're full, and when to stop. You naturally eat less and feel satisfied more. Fat is also the food of your hormonal system, so upping your fat intake first thing in the morning can readily turn hormonal chaos into hormonal harmony.

All this being said, not all fats are created equal. What's the high-quality fat on Chef Marcella's menu?

You might not like what I'm about to say: I am a *huge fan* of saturated fats from pastured, humanely raised animals: butter, ghee, chicken schmaltz, lard (yes, lard), duck fat, and beef tallow. These sacred substances, widely condemned as morally reprehensible, are among the most satisfying foods you can give your brain, your belly, and your entire nervous system. Imagine your hormones soaking in a deliciously warm bath, and you have some glimpse of the power of saturated fats.

If you're not ready or inclined to praise the lard as I do, I invite you to explore appreciatively the monounsaturated plant fats that are likewise wonderful and available: olives, avocadoes, coconut, macadamia nuts, and so on. Even if you don't eat fat for lunch or supper, at least have some at breakfast, so your metabolism starts the day on a tank of high-octane fuel.

Protein

We do not lack for protein in our industrialized diets, but most of us reserve high-protein foods for suppertime. When you eat a twenty-four-ounce steak for dinner and then head to the La-Z-Boy for some channel surfing, most of that protein is going to waste, because the body can use only so much at one time.

Try eating your protein in the morning instead, to give your body and belly and brain fuel to burn and feel satisfied with. Among its many benefits, protein helps build lean muscle mass, so eating an abundance of protein—nuts, beans, cheese, eggs, meat—at the start of your day, when your body has enough time to utilize it fully, will help you both feel fuller longer and burn fat more efficiently.

Fiber

Also known by the charmed, antiquated name of *roughage,* fiber for breakfast slows down the rush of glucose into the blood stream, creates a feeling of fullness and satisfaction with your food, helps your brain and belly know when enough is enough, and blesses you with blissful regularity.

Don't be fooled by "high fiber" processed breakfast cereals, breakfast bars, or energy bars. Always, when buying a packaged food product, look carefully at the ingredients before you purchase. Turn the package around and read the small print. If you see anything that resembles sugar in the first five ingredients—including *fructose, dextrose, corn syrup,* and so on—just walk away, Renée. Sugar in any form is not your friend first thing in the morning. Reach instead for multigrain breakfast cereals with just the grains and nothing more. Or skip the grains altogether and get your fiber from beans, nuts, seeds, and vegetables.

Chef Marcella's Favorite Breakfasts

Putting these together, breakfast *á la Marcella* looks like the following. Try your own combinations to see what works for you:

- poached eggs over sautéed greens and mushrooms
- black beans and sprouted-grain tortillas with avocado, cilantro, and salsa
- broiled fish with miso soup, sea veggies, and lacto-fermented pickles
- sprouted-grain sourdough toast schmeared with any combination of goat cheese, hummus, hard-boiled eggs, sardines, tomato, avocado, herbs, greens, and sprouts
- *congee* (brown rice porridge) with chicken, egg drop, greens, and mushrooms
- savory multigrain breakfast cereal with butter, *tamari* (naturally fermented soy sauce), toasted nuts or seeds, and sautéed greens.

Chef Marcella also loves supper for breakfast. If you're in a time pinch in the morning, warm up some of last night's dinner. Soups and stews, in particular, are wonderfully nourishing and hydrating supports to get your metabolic motor humming. Plus, they're often much tastier the day after they're made, when the flavors have had a chance to really get to know each other.

Motivational giant Tony Robbins once said that the most effective changes are not big ones. They're usually a one-millimeter shift.[5] Eating a nourishing breakfast every day can be that one-millimeter habit that swings your life from hopeless to happy.

Commit to eating a hearty, savory breakfast every day for seven days. If that works, commit to another seven. If you get stuck, tap it out. And hang in there! You deserve the nourishment you desire.

Let's Do Some Tapping

Say the following statement to yourself: "Each day, I enjoy nourishing myself with a complete and delicious breakfast." How true does that feel, with 100 percent being absolute truth? Tune into any body sensations, emotions, story lines, or self-talk that comes up. If your number feels low, and resistance is high, use the following Tapping guide to tune into what's in the way. Change the words as you need. See what comes up:

Tapping Guide 9.1: Eating a Good Breakfast

SETUP STATEMENT: *Even though I struggle with eating a good breakfast, I deeply and completely love and accept myself.* (Say aloud one to three times.)

Top of the head: *Eating breakfast—*

Eyebrow: *It's too much work.*

Side of the eye: *I don't have time.*

Under the eye: *I can't get it together to make a good breakfast.*

Under the nose: *It feels overwhelming even to try.*

Under the mouth: *People like me don't eat a good breakfast.*

Collarbone: *I've never had a good breakfast.*

Under arm: *Why start now?*

Top of the head: *It's easier to just skip it.*

Eyebrow: *Maybe I don't deserve that much nourishment.*

Side of the eye: *It's easier to deny my need for breakfast.*

Under the eye: *I can't take care of myself like that.*

Under the nose: *It's way too healthy to eat a good breakfast.*

Under the mouth: *People like me aren't healthy with food.*

Collarbone: *Fuhgeddaboudit.*

Under arm: *Just give me some coffee and doughnuts.*

Top of the head: *I wonder why I have so much resistance.*

Eyebrow: *Why do I resist nurturing myself?*

Side of the eye: *I wonder what that's about—*

Under the eye: *This resistance I feel to breakfast,*

Under the nose: *And other ways of taking care of myself.*

Under the mouth: *I own it completely.*

Collarbone: *And I'm open to changing it.*

Under arm: *I wonder what that change would feel like.*

Top of the head: *What if I ate a good breakfast every day?*

Eyebrow: *And felt better throughout the day?*

Side of the eye: *And didn't have to crave and binge?*

Under the eye: *Can I step into this?*

Under the nose: *Is it okay?*

Under the mouth: *I don't know.*

Collarbone: *But I'm open to it and willing to explore it.*

Under arm: *And I love myself for that willingness.*

Take a nice deep breath. Check in with your initial distress level—is it higher, lower, or about the same? Keep repeating rounds of Tapping until you feel relief.

If breakfast feels hard because being in the kitchen at all freaks you out, tune in to the following chapter, where I'll take your hand and reintroduce you to the best room in your home.

To tap along with audio recordings of this and other Tapping guides, visit www. marcellafriel.com/taptasteheal.

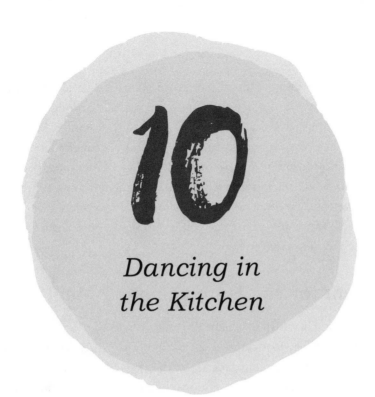

10

Dancing in the Kitchen

In the circles I run in and market to, the home-cooked meal is revered as the ultimate expression of food integrity. [It] indicates a reverence for our bodies' fuel, a respect for biology, and a committed remedial spirit toward all the shenanigans in our industrial, pathogen-laden, nutrient-deficient food-and-farming system.

—JOEL SALATIN

IN MODERN SOCIETY, we are confronting an unprecedented dilemma. On the one hand, procuring food has never been easier. Unlike our ancestors who had to spear the wooly mammoth or till stubborn earth for a single turnip, we have restaurants, drive-throughs, and cafeterias preparing more food than we could ever consume. With nothing more than a word, a click, or a scan, our victuals appear magically before us.

Yet we're still hungry.

It's not that our distended bellies growl as we stare glassy-eyed at an empty bowl. We long for deeper nourishment than takeout can provide. We long for home-cooked meals eaten with those we love.

The meal table is the fulcrum of human civilization. Our capacity to cook food is one of the behaviors that distinguish us from other animals. Sharing food is how we first learn to become relational. Whether the fare is tasty or terrible, knowing those who prepared it, sitting at the table with them, making eye contact, and engaging in conversation provide sustenance that mere caloric intake cannot supply.

And while we might feel diffident about home cooking, we subconsciously miss it as we open take-out cartons, eat at our desks, or graze mindlessly. We mourn its loss as we ruefully watch family members chow down microwaved meals while checking social media.

Requiem for the Home-Cooked Meal

According to food historian Laura Shapiro,[1] after World War II, the military food-production technology that churned out K-rations for hungry troops was turned to civilian use, producing canned meats, freeze-dried coffee, dehydrated potatoes, powdered orange juice, and other products. The processed food industry heavily marketed its goods to housewives, telling them to regard home cooking as drudgery and seducing them with these "sophisticated" instant foods.

Initially, however, women didn't like the taste of these new creations; nor did they like not cooking. The industry responded by fashioning convenience foods that required the preparer to perform at least one faux-cooking action: "add milk to special sauce packet" or "beat one egg into cake mix."

As the 1960s unfolded, the food industry began portraying home cooking as tantamount to domestic slavery at the same time that women were migrating *en masse* from the kitchen stove to the office desk. Capitalizing on this demographic shift, the industry promoted processed convenience foods as allies of women's liberation.

Now, nearly half a century later, the home-cooked meal has gone the way of the rotary-dial telephone: a quaint relic of a slower past. But the fallout of that loss is neither quaint nor charming.

Why Home Cooking Matters

Food journalist Michael Pollan points out that we Americans spend an average of twenty-seven minutes per day on meal preparation—and most of that involves heating a can of soup or microwaving a frozen pizza. Our favorite meal, for both lunch and dinner, is a sandwich and a soda.[2]

We widely regard cooking as an obstacle to the rest of our life, our chief complaint being that it takes too much time. (Yet since the beginning of the twenty-first century, we've miraculously found an extra three and a half hours a day to surf the internet.[3]) As the time spent in food preparation has fallen, calorie consumption has risen. It's no secret that processed foods are laden with refined sugars, rancid fats, and excess sodium. We're so rife with cancer, diabetes, and other degenerative diseases that we've come to regard them as normal occurrences in human life.

Allowing corporations to cook for us has not only made us fatter and sicker. The loss of home cooking and community meals, combined with other factors, has plunged us into a life-threatening epidemic of alienation. As renowned cardiologist Dean Ornish puts it, "There isn't any other factor in medicine … that has a greater impact on our quality of life, incidence of illness and premature death from all causes than loneliness and isolation."[4]

What Is a Meal, Anyway?

Beyond an occasional pedicure, how many of us invest our time in activities that demonstrate real, substantive self-care? Planning, preparing, and eating a truly nourishing meal are some of those activities. If we never register mentally the experience of sitting down and eating a full meal, we regard everything we eat as a "snack," or "something on the go," which then gives us a false reason to eat more later. Thus we overeat without ever truly eating. We are, in author Raj Patel's words, "stuffed and starved."[5] We consume a surfeit of calories so nutritionally bankrupt that they leave us malnourished. (And if that's the condition of our body, what does that say about the condition of our soul?)

What is a meal? A meal is a ritual that takes time, much like slow lovemaking. If attention is indeed the highest form of love, serving a meal to yourself and your loved ones is a humble offering that elevates everyday life to a cause for celebration.

As meditation master Chögyam Trungpa pointed out, "The extension of your sanity and your dignity may depend on how you use your fork."[6] To set a table, gather loved ones, and share a meal—such gestures are small deposits in the cosmic bank account of love. They return dividends of joy and affirm that life—of itself, by itself—is worthy of such offerings.

Meals are most commonly eaten sitting down, either in one's own company or in the company of loved ones. The food, typically prepared from scratch, is served on dishes that do require dishwashing cleanup but spares Mother Earth from having to bear more of our litter load.

A meal has components to it, typically a protein source of some kind along with a complex carbohydrate and some vegetables. When you finish a meal, you feel complete, replete, satisfied, free of craving, and fully fed. Your body says thank you and happily sets about its work of turning that food into nourishment.

Snacks, by contrast, are usually prepackaged cheap foods, eaten alone, while multitasking, with all packaging carelessly tossed into the trash. After snacking, the belly says, "You want me to turn *this* into health for you? Sorry, sweetheart. You're outta luck."

Perhaps I'm getting on my soapbox here. And yes, some snacks can be health supportive, such as nuts or dried fruit. And some of us need those boosters to keep our blood sugar stable during the day, which keeps us from reaching for the "harder stuff." And that's great, no doubt.

But still—aren't you worth one home-cooked meal a day? Or maybe even a few a week? Or an all-day cookfest on Sunday that supplies the meals for half of the next week? Think about it: what would be the payoff of one less hour on Facebook to nourish the flesh of your flesh and the blood of your blood? Now that I've seduced you into the kitchen—will you dance with me?

Celebrating Everyday Life at the Meal Table

If you're someone who has steered clear of the kitchen all your life, my soft suggestion to you is to allow yourself to be a beginner. Be willing to fumble and bumble and make mistakes. In the reassuring words of Zen chef Edward Espe Brown, "Who says you can't cook? I give you permission. You can look with your eyes and feel with your hands, smell with your nose, and taste with your tongue. You can think and create, be inspired, or stumble along. You keep finding your way."[7]

Where do we start with the seemingly monumental task of regularly cooking nourishing meals at home? If you already feel overwhelmed, you can just jump to the Tapping guide at the end of this chapter. Otherwise, here are a few ideas that even a beginner can start to apply:

> *Learn to cook at least one food well,* whether it's steaming green beans, roasting a potato, or panfrying a chicken thigh. You don't have to mimic the gladiatorial spectacle of television cooking shows. Simple is good enough.

❧ *Bring ordinary celebrations into cooking and eating.* Listen to relaxing music. Clear and set the table, even if it's only for you. (In the early episodes of *The French Chef,* Julia Child always sat down alone at a set table to eat her own creations.)

❧ *Eat with others whenever possible.* Plan at least one night a week for a family supper. If you live alone, invite a friend to eat with you. We eat in a more civilized fashion when we eat with others.

❧ *Learn the difference between whole foods and processed foods.* Flip back to chapter 8 to refresh your memory if you're a bit rusty.

❧ *Create your own food rituals.* Eat from a beautiful bowl. Teach your children to wash their own napkins. Learn a meal chant or create one of your own.

Chef Marcella's Tips for Easy Meal Planning

Take time. Make the kitchen a sacred space for meal prep. Consider deeply the food to be prepared, the ingredients to be gathered, the timing of the cooking, and the guests to be fed. This is your chance to make love with your food. Give it all you got, and let me know how it goes.

The Basics

My model meal is not far from the old-fashioned meat-potatoes-and-vegetables menu that was so popular in the Mom-cooks-at-home 1950s. Despite its fuddy-duddy image, it remains a good blueprint and lends itself to lots of diversity.

I first look at the "meat"—the main protein source in the meal. The word *protein* means "primary substance" and gives credence to the saying "You are what you eat." It is the centerpiece of the meal. What will it be? Fowl, fish, red meat, white meat, beans, eggs, or dairy foods? The first point of meal planning in Chef Marcella's kitchen is always to identify the protein.

Then I look at the "potatoes," which, in reality, means *complex carbohydrates.* These include starchy vegetables (sweet potatoes, carrots, parsnips, turnips, rutabagas, celery root, winter squash, and so on) or whole grains (brown rice, quinoa, millet, buckwheat, and corn meal). What foods are filling that function?

The vegetables include whatever is in season and appropriate to the region. I eat religiously from farmers' markets and private gardens; in the off-season, I rely on whatever local, seasonal produce I can find.

In my day-to-day cooking, I prepare foods simply but have top-notch condiments on hand, such as flavored oils, infused vinegars, gourmet salts and peppers, prepared spice mixes, and fancy mustards. These luxurious extras quickly take a meal from ordinary to extraordinary. Douse a roasted sweet potato with truffle oil and smoked salt; toss some cut cauliflower with a curry spice blend and panfry in ghee or coconut oil; drizzle barrel-aged balsamic vinegar over steamed green beans. The cooking is simple—roasting, frying, steaming—the garnishing more elaborate. Get the picture?

As I sit at a desk most of my workday, my favorite food ritual when eating solo is to prepare a one-bowl meal and eat sitting cross-legged on my sofa. I find no need to be too table-and-chairs stuffy about mindful eating. My desire is to make my body comfy. I also eat outdoors as much as I can in warm weather.

Beyond the Basics

There are a number of factors I pay attention to include in meals:

- *Colors:* There's a Japanese saying, *me de taberu,*[8] or "one eats first with the eyes." I look at my plate before I eat. Is the meal visually appealing? Is there a diversity of color? Black beans, yellow corn, red roasted peppers, white sour cream, green avocado, even greener cilantro? "Eating the rainbow" is the best way to ensure that I'm getting all the macro- and micronutrients I need.

- *Textures:* Do I have a nice mix of creamy, crunchy, chewy, crispy? Do I have both starchy and non-starchy foods? How about a bowl of miso soup with chewy buckwheat soba noodles, crunchy carrot slivers, slippery wilted spinach, and dense fish?

- *Flavors:* A well-balanced meal contains myriad flavors: sweet, salty, sour, bitter, pungent, and astringent. Would you like a red curry with chicken, ginger, cauliflower, and potatoes; a side dish of cucumber *raita* (yogurt condiment); plus some crispy lentil crackers *(papadum)* and lime pickle? Yowza! How many flavors can you identify in that one meal?

- *Something Raw:* No matter what time of year I'm eating, I always include some raw foods to get those life-affirming enzymes. I'm not a fan of salads in winter, but I will garnish a heartily cooked lamb stew with freshly grated carrots and turnips.

ஃ *Something Fermented:* And it wouldn't be a Chef Marcella meal if it didn't include something fermented: a forkful of sauerkraut, a dollop of yogurt or crème fraiche, or some lacto-fermented veggies to round out the meal and give the digestion a little extra support.

Dancing in the Kitchen

Finally, to make the cooking experience as enjoyable as possible, I'm always sure to

ஃ change into comfy clothes,

ஃ put on a fun or sexy apron,

ஃ play some pleasant music or listen to an interesting audiobook,

ஃ clear the dinner table of bills and other distractions and use it only for eating, and

ஃ invite others to join me, if that's relaxing (or if I'd prefer, keep the space all to myself).

What would make you feel yummy when you eat your meal? Would you enjoy the Zen simplicity of modest, home-cooked fare for one? Or do you need to lie on your divan and have your beloved feed you one delicious morsel at a time? (Remember, the Universe says *yes* to every thought. Even if you don't have it yet, ask, and it shall be given.)

The Banquet in the First Bite

Once your meal is in front of you, pause for a moment before digging in. Place one or both hands on your heart and take three deep, conscious breaths. Allow your mind to settle into your heart center until you feel a slight separation from the concerns of the day.

Then bring all your attention to your food. Notice the colors, textures, shapes, and smells. What do you observe? How does your body feel in relation to this food?

Take a few more deep breaths. Bring one bite of food to your mouth. Be as fully present to that first bite as you can. What is your mouth saying about this food? What is your stomach saying? What other sensations are arising?

Continue eating, bringing your attention back to the act of eating when it wants to go elsewhere. How does your experience change as you eat? Can you find the point when your body says, "Enough"?

Don't worry about doing this perfectly. Just show up with your sincere desire to heal, and you will, with repeated practice, come to a place of deep appreciation for the meal in front of you, however imperfect it—or you—might be.

Let's Do Some Tapping

Now that I have sung the praises of reclaiming the sacred art of home cooking, I also recognize that, for some of you, the kitchen isn't such a fun place to be. The kitchen might be utterly alien territory or, worse, a place of trauma. The kitchen might have been the place where Mom first put you on a diet or labeled you a klutz for sending the mixing bowl crashing to the floor. Or maybe it was at the meal table that you had to endure all of Grandpa's icky remarks about your body in the presence of other family members.

If this is the case, I want to invite you, as best as you can in this moment, to take a few deep breaths and acknowledge fully whatever un-okay stuff went on in the kitchens of your past. You might want to pull out your journal and jot down some thoughts about what happened, what you've made those experiences mean about yourself and others, and what obstacles you currently experience as a result of those circumstances.

You might then want to tap along with the following Tapping guide.

Tapping Guide 10.1: "I'm Not Comfortable in the Kitchen"

SETUP STATEMENT: *Even though I don't feel comfortable in the kitchen, I deeply love and accept myself.* (Say aloud one to three times.)

Top of the head: *I'm not comfortable in the kitchen.*

Eyebrow: *I'm just not at home there.*

Side of the eye: *I don't feel comfortable at all.*

Under the eye: *I'd just as soon avoid the kitchen.*

Under the nose: *It's really uncomfortable to be in there.*

Under the mouth: *Trying to do anything—*

Collarbone: *It's too painful.*

Under arm: *I'd rather avoid the kitchen.*

Top of the head: *I don't want to be reminded of what I feel*

Eyebrow: *When I'm in the kitchen.*

Side of the eye: *I don't want to face it.*

Under the eye: *I wish there were some way around it—*

Under the nose: *All this discomfort I feel,*

Under the mouth: *And everything it means to me.*

Collarbone: *As best I can in this moment,*

Under arm: *I choose to be kind to myself.*

Top of the head: *I give myself lots of understanding.*

Eyebrow: *It's okay.*

Side of the eye: *Feeling so uneasy in the kitchen—*

Under the eye: *I give it lots of room to be.*

Under the nose: *Nothing to fix or change—*

Under the mouth: *Just acknowledging and accepting,*

Collarbone: *Giving it space,*

Under arm: *Giving myself lots of understanding.*

Top of the head: *All this discomfort I feel—*

Eyebrow: *And everything it means to me—*

Side of the eye: *It's okay for it to just be here.*

Under the eye: *It's okay for me to relax.*

Under the nose: *It's okay for me to feel how I feel.*

Under the mouth: *I totally own this is where I'm at.*

Collarbone: *And I love myself unconditionally,*

Under arm: *Exactly as I am in this moment.*

Take a nice deep breath. Check in with your initial distress level—is it higher, lower, or about the same? Keep repeating rounds of Tapping until you feel relief.

If you know how much better the quality of your life would be if you ate more home-cooked food but still feel resistance to incorporating that practice into your life, then tap along right here in Tapping guide 10.2.

Tapping Guide 10.2: "I Hate Cooking"

SETUP STATEMENT: *Even though I hate cooking, I deeply and completely love and accept myself. (Say aloud one to three times.)*

Top of the head: *I hate cooking.*

Eyebrow: *I can't help it—I just hate it.*

Side of the eye: *It's the last thing I ever want to do.*

Under the eye: *I'm just not interested in cooking.*

Under the nose: *I really hate it.*

Under the mouth: *And I can't imagine I could ever enjoy it.*

Collarbone: *And that's just where I'm at.*

Under arm: *I totally own it.*

Top of the head: *I can't be bothered.*

Eyebrow: *But then again, I don't eat very well.*

Side of the eye: *If I don't eat home-cooked food,*

Under the eye: *I'm living on restaurants and takeout—*

Under the nose: *Not a great option.*

Under the mouth: *But I really hate to cook.*

Collarbone: *So what can I do?*

Under arm: *I feel pretty stuck.*

Top of the head: *I wonder why I hate it so much.*

Eyebrow: *When did I first start hating to cook?*

Side of the eye: *I wonder where that set in—*

Under the eye: *All this resistance I feel to cooking.*

Under the nose: *I wonder what it's about.*

Under the mouth: *What would I find if I became curious?*

Collarbone: *I wonder what's beneath the resistance.*

Under arm: *What could it be?*

Top of the head: *Whatever it is,*

Eyebrow: *Maybe I can't open up to cooking today,*

Side of the eye: *But I'm willing to be open*

Under the eye: *To a different experience of cooking.*

Under the nose: *I'm willing to experience something new.*

Under the mouth: *I'm willing to trade in my old story*

Collarbone: *And take a fresh start.*

Under arm: *And I totally love myself for that.*

Take a nice deep breath. Check in with your initial distress level—is it higher, lower, or about the same? Keep repeating rounds of Tapping until you feel relief.

To tap along with audio recordings of this and other Tapping guides, visit www.marcellafriel.com/taptasteheal.

11

"Can I Love Myself Even with This?"

It's only when we alter our eating habits out of love and respect for ourselves that lasting change has any real chance to take root in our lives.

—KATHERINE WOODWARD THOMAS

"I'VE GAINED TEN pounds in the last two weeks. I'm so disappointed in myself. I should be over this by now."

These were the words of my client Linda. They were nothing new. After listening to her bemoan her body condition, I asked, "Linda, I wonder if your true addiction is not to the food but to the disappointment? Might you be using your food behaviors to maintain your story of being disappointed in yourself?"

Linda fell silent but was open to my suggestion. I asked her to close her eyes, place a hand on her heart, take a few deep breaths, and tell me all the things she genuinely loved and appreciated about herself. She free-associated while I took notes.

I sent her my notes after our session, along with the suggestion that she audio-record her proclamation of self-appreciation and listen to it every morning upon awakening. "This feels good," she texted me the following day. "I really like it!"

There's Nothing Wrong with You

If you are struggling to heal your relationship with food, it's seductive to feel, deep down, that something is horribly wrong with you and to believe that, if you punish yourself enough by eating celery sticks instead of cookies, you'll one day reach that ever-elusive promised land of a "perfect" diet and "perfect" body weight. When you inevitably fail to meet such tyrannical expectations, you turn the blame inward and double down on the celery sticks—at least until the next binge.

In this chapter, I want to take you beyond just losing the weight or quitting the sugar for good. Let me share with you my secret recipe for the most profound, enduring, and rewarding tool you can ever use for transforming your struggles into blessings at the deepest level of your being. Ready? Let's begin.

What It Takes to Heal

When I was a natural-foods culinary instructor, one of my favorite classes to teach was Therapeutic Menu Planning—how to prepare health-supportive menu plans for those who suffer from cancer, diabetes, obesity, and other chronic health hindrances.

I always began the class by asking students, "What does it actually mean to heal something? Is *healing* a disease the same as *curing* it? Can someone be cured of a disease but not healed? Can someone be healed but not cured?"

As we batted around our ideas, words such as *wholeness* and *integration* and *alignment* ended up on the whiteboard. I would then invite them to explore what's at the *root* of attaining wholeness or integration or alignment. They would often look at me quizzically while pondering the possibilities.

In our take-a-pill-and-feel-better culture, *curing*—or symptom relief—is the apogee of recovery from illness. But while symptom relief is certainly desirable, it is not, in and of itself, the optimal outcome. What is it, then, that heals any disease or malaise at its root?

Forgiveness.

For those of us who struggle with food, the quest for healing can be a maddening maze of diet plans and exercise regimens fueled by a multi-billion-dollar diet industry that wants to keep us buying the next meal-replacement products or fitness gadgetry. None of it will ever create lasting change.

The key to choosing your food with self-love versus self-loathing and making lifelong friends with your body is forgiveness. Forgiveness appeases all those stress hormones we talked about a few chapters ago. It calms our state of mind, which, in turn, alleviates the triggers that cause the body to crave food and hold on to excess weight. So when you forgive, you lose both emotional and physical pounds.

A Different View of Forgiveness

Unless we have the fortitude of Mother Teresa, forgiveness for most of us is pretty tough. In one of his Sunday sermons, Pastor Rob Koke at Shoreline Christian Church in Austin, Texas, unpacked some common misbeliefs that can hamper our efforts to forgive:

> Forgiveness is not taking the blame ourselves. It's not earned or deserved because somebody pacifies us. It is not getting even, it's not feeling sympathy, it's not trying to be nice. It is not becoming a weak doormat.

> Forgiveness is erasing the offense, cutting off the debt. It's to release an account that's due; it's to wipe the slate clean. Forgive as you have been forgiven.[1]

Merriam-Webster has two simple definitions of *forgive:* "to cease to feel resentment," and "to grant relief from payment."[2] If you contemplate these definitions in relation to each other, you might see what Pastor Rob is saying: our emotions are a form of currency.

When we hold on to a grievance, it's like jacking up our credit cards. We're paying the energy bill on our previous emotional expenditures in order to keep resentment, anger, and victimization alive. As that debt increases over time, we pay usurious late fees and interest rates in addictions and degenerative disease. Eventually, we default into *spiritual bankruptcy* as our soul calcifies into shame, bitterness, regret, and so forth.

Forgiveness, then, is bringing our emotional currency into present time. When we genuinely forgive, we release the expectation that we will feel better once we make people, places, and circumstances conform to our expectations of how they should have been or should be now. In doing so, we cash in the "you-owe-me" attitude of *justice* and invest in a wealthier vision of *peace* that acknowledges things as they are.

For forgiveness to be genuine, before we even think of forgiving another, we must first venture into our own dark side. We must find and befriend the parts of ourselves we have split off, denied, or neglected. We must call our spirit home from those we believe to be the cause of our suffering. We must unmask the monsters of our soul to discover the keys to liberation that they've been holding for us all along.

Ultimately, true forgiveness is tantamount to death. We must die to our old story of what happened, who hurt us, and how we are flawed. We are then reborn in the light of our true nature. This is why forgiveness is so hard. It's not that we don't want to forgive; it's that we can't bear the brilliance of who we become once we do.

Release the Banana

The Second Noble Truth of Buddhism states that we suffer because we hold on. Like the classic story of the monkey that would rather die than let go of the banana in the box-trap, we perversely find it easier to hold on to toxic resentments than to release and forgive.

This is not our fault. As medical intuitive Caroline Myss points out, we, as a culture, have become addicted to the eye-for-an-eye mentality. If someone harms us, we believe resolution will come when the perpetrators have paid the penalty for their actions. Justice, however, is only a partial solution. Justice alone does not give us peace and often leaves us still smoldering even after the price has been paid.[3]

For women, forgiveness is especially problematic, as we are conditioned to be peacemakers and pressured to forgive quickly in the interest of being "nice." We also bear the burden of social conditioning to be sweet, pretty, and helpful to others. We are told to never look bad, smell bad, raise our voices, get in the way, or—heaven forbid—upset anyone.

As a result, we have endured and internalized the neuroses of our ancestors and the degradation of our culture. We felt our mother's projected shame when she put us on a diet at age eight and obsessed over every detail of our appearance. We absorbed Dad's misogyny in the salacious remarks he made about female bodies, including our own. We cringed at the violence of skinny-girl images paraded before us, knowing that our big-boned frame could never shrink down to that impossible size. And we reveled in the desperate pleasure of chips, cookies, chocolate, ice cream—our best and only friends when all else failed.

Having few or no reference points outside that insanity, we drove the madness inward and made it about us. We confused our food struggle with our value as a human being. From that confusion, we forged a fragmented identity of ourselves as unworthy, flawed, and condemned.

Forgiveness, then, begins with detaching ourselves first from our own insanity and then from the madness of those around us. As we meet and embrace those un-sweet and un-pretty parts of ourselves and release the shame that lurks in our shadows, we realize that Mother's shaming was more about her insecurity than our appearance. We get that Dad would have made those rude remarks about any young woman, and it had nothing to do with us. We recognize that our true beauty emanates naturally from the sparkle of our self-esteem and has nothing to do with our dress size.

What Does It Take to Forgive?

I hope you're getting the picture that, more than a quick "I'm sorry" or "It's okay," true forgiveness is a journey of the soul. Every genuine spiritual tradition has powerful teachings for cultivating forgiveness. If you belong to such a tradition, I invite you to refresh your connection to those practices, if it's gotten rusty. You can also borrow some ingredients from Chef Marcella's forgiveness pantry and add them to your own mix:

1. *Start where you are.* Don't try to be a forgiveness superhero right out of the gate. The best starting point is to touch and be lovingly patient with those shadow parts of yourself that have kept you stuck in your pain. Forgiveness comes in its own time and will most likely come sooner if you accept yourself where you are.

2. *Don't rush or figure out forgiveness.* Forgiveness is a spiritual process that doesn't answer to logic. When we make a genuine decision to forgive, our inner and outer worlds shape-shift around our intention. We must set our thinking aside to allow the path to unfold in its own perfect way.

3. *Allow another to witness your pain.* However wise we are spiritually, we cannot heal our pain without support from others. Even if we can identify the origins of our struggles with food, we can't liberate ourselves using the brain that got us into our predicament to begin with. When you are ready, disclose your wounds to someone you can trust. Ideally, this person has

overcome their own ordeals and can provide guidance, tools, and emotional support that will catapult your forgiveness forward.

4. *Let it all out.* Don't be spiritually hygienic while unpacking your pain. The more rage, pettiness, ugliness, and nastiness you can disgorge, the faster the healing.

5. *Know that forgiveness takes many forms.* You might forgive someone and never want to talk to them again. You might need to set new terms for the relationship. It's okay to set whatever boundaries you need for your healing. True forgiveness requires a heroic and willing heart. It doesn't always look nice-nice.

Which Practices Support Forgiveness?

If you're ready for some nuts-and-bolts tools to help you forgive, here are a few practices that I have collaged together from various spiritual traditions. You can do any one of these or all three in succession. You can do these alone or with a witness. (If you do them alone, I suggest you "bookend" them with someone: contact that person beforehand and describe what you intend to do; then contact them again afterward to recount the experience.)

The Resentment Buster

This is a powerful practice if rage, righteous anger, and other strong emotions hamper your ability to forgive.

Write a letter to the person you're trying to forgive, whether yourself or someone else, venting all your grievances and negativity. Don't make sense, don't be spiritual, and definitely don't be nice. This letter is for your eyes only. (If your emotions are particularly raw, use the Tapping guide at the end of this chapter to process them more quickly.)

When you feel complete, imagine yourself as that person and write a letter from them back to you. Allow them to express all their raw emotions and judgments about you. Again, no nice-nice. This is an all-out smackdown.

Continue writing back and forth in this way until the negativity is exhausted on both sides. This could take hours, days, or weeks. Give yourself as much time as you need without procrastinating.

When the negativity feels like it's been discharged on both sides, write a letter of appreciation from you to that person. Express whatever goodwill and kind regards that you can. Write a letter from that person back to you expressing those same feelings. Keep writing back and forth until the process feels complete. Read them aloud to yourself (or to someone else, if that feels okay); then burn or compost the letters.

The Decision Ritual

You'll need a candle, a journal, and, if you have one, a photograph of the person you want to forgive. You'll also need a private space, free from interruption. Plan to spend at least thirty minutes performing this ritual.

> Light your candle.
>
> Begin by sitting in meditation with your eyes closed and your hands on your heart, connecting to your heartbeat. If your attention wanders, bring it back to that beating heart. Sit this way until you feel more settled in your awareness.
>
> If you have a photo of the person, allow yourself to gaze at it, without thinking of anything in particular. Notice the details of the photo, especially the look on that person's face and their body posture. When you're ready, spend a few minutes journaling about why you want to forgive this person. If it feels hard to forgive, write about that.
>
> When your writing is complete, say to the photo, "[Name], I now forgive you."

Repeat this aloud until you feel complete. Spend a few moments being present to the thoughts and feelings that arise. If they're particularly strong, use the Tapping guide at the end of this chapter to move the energy through.

The Fourteen-Day Prayer

In the *Big Book of Alcoholics Anonymous,* a recovering drunk shares pearls of wisdom on the power of this practice:

> If you have a resentment you want to be free of, if you will pray for the person or the thing that you resent, you will be free. If you will ask in prayer for everything you want for yourself to be given to them, you will be free. Ask for their health, their prosperity, their happiness, and you will

be free. Even when you don't really want it for them, and your prayers are only words and you don't mean it, go ahead and do it anyway. Do it every day for two weeks, and you will find you have come to mean it and to want it for them, and you will realize that where you used to feel bitterness and resentment and hatred, you now feel compassion and love.[4]

Every day, for fourteen days, pray—in whatever way prayer shows up for you—for the person you'd like to forgive. Begin by reflecting on what you seek to gain from forgiving that person (peace, joy, relief, freedom). Arouse those feelings in your heart. You might want to say aloud to yourself, "May I, [your name], be happy. May I be well. May I be joyful. May I be free." Give those feelings to yourself as best you can. Then mentally give those feelings away to the other person, saying, "[name], may you be happy. May you be peaceful. May you be joyful. May you be free." (If you like, you can extend it out to everyone: "May all beings be happy …" and so on.)

If the object of your forgiveness is still alive, don't be surprised if something in the relationship profoundly shifts as a result of this practice. That person might write an actual letter to you, offer a heartfelt apology, or just start being a kinder person. If you hold the view that, on the quantum level, we are all truly one, you must likewise hold space for the potential impact your act of forgiveness can have on others.

The Most Abiding Forgiveness

My client Tammy was making terrific progress with her food but was still seized with anxiety whenever she had lunch with her girlfriends. While the ladies blithely ordered their fare, Tammy obsessed over the menu, pitting what she wanted against what she "should" have.

When we looked into the energetic roots of this struggle, Tammy saw herself as a teenage mom, watching her girlfriends having fun while she was swamped with a low-functioning husband and two young daughters. Tammy remembered glumly looking on at her high-school graduation while her classmates received awards and tossed their caps in the air.

I guided Tammy through a Tapping meditation in which she journeyed back in time to soothe and reassure her younger self, then reenvisioned the graduation experience so that she walked her inner teenager onto the stage and awarded her—to a standing ovation—a certificate of thanks for blessing the planet with two beautiful children. Self-forgiveness flooded through Tammy as she imagined this new scenario. Weeks later she excitedly reported, "I eat whatever I want now. And by the way, I've lost fifteen pounds! It's slow, it's nothing dramatic, and that's just fine with me."

While we might well have people and circumstances in our lives that have indeed harmed us, our first, last, and most abiding forgiveness is to ourselves. Freeing ourselves from our compulsive food behaviors, then, is not about white-knuckling our way through punitive abstinence, eating lettuce when we really want to face-plant in an ice-cream sundae. It's about releasing everything we have made those behaviors mean about us. It's not about going on the next Grapefruit Diet but rather about letting go of being someone who needs to diet to begin with. Forgiveness entails saying these truths to ourselves and having them said to us over and over, until they take root in our cell tissue:

> ❧ "Your struggles with food are not your fault. They have been your best way of loving yourself in difficult circumstances."
>
> ❧ "You are not your traumas."
>
> ❧ "There is nothing wrong with you or bad about you. You are an amazing being, exactly as you are."

These truths are the stepping stones by which the broken fragments of our soul come tiptoeing home to stay. We re-collect ourselves, re-member ourselves, and, in so doing, realize in our very core that, ultimately, nothing was ever out of place. We see with bird's-eye-view clarity that there never was, fundamentally, a problem. There have just been things in the way that are moved out of the way as we choose to allow them to be.

As that realization washes away whatever vestiges of shame we had been harboring, our addiction, once our worst enemy, becomes the teacher that shows us the goodness of our heart that was never tarnished to begin with. The healing we have been seeking all these years flows through us like a mighty river that never runs dry.

Does this mean you miraculously live happily ever after? Well, no. It's more that, when faced with your old patterns, you can ask yourself the question my late friend Ellen asked herself at each stage of her cancer journey:

"Can I love myself, even with this?"

Let's Do Some Tapping

What would your life—and your food—be like if you could say, "I deeply love and accept myself," and *mean it?*

Place your hands on your heart and take three deep breaths. Say aloud to yourself, "I deeply love and completely forgive myself in this moment." See what comes up and tap on that. If you want to extend forgiveness to yourself but find your forgiveness muscle is in spasm, tap along with the following Tapping guide to help that muscle loosen up and relax.

Begin by tuning in to the reasons why you find it hard to forgive yourself. If there are no specific circumstances connected to your inability to forgive, then tune in to the general feeling of being unable to allow yourself to experience your own goodness of being. See if there's a place in your body where that lack of forgiveness resides.

Tapping Guide 11.1: "I Can't Forgive Myself"

SETUP STATEMENT: *Even though I find it really hard to forgive myself, I choose to forgive myself anyway.* (Say aloud one to three times.)

Top of the head: *I refuse to forgive myself.*

Eyebrow: *I absolutely refuse to forgive myself.*

Side of the eye: *There's no way I deserve forgiveness.*

Under the eye: *I can't accept that I could deserve forgiveness.*

Under the nose: *How could someone like me deserve forgiveness?*

Under the mouth: *I'm such a bad person.*

Collarbone: *I've done horrible things that can't be forgiven.*

Under arm: *I'm the worst of the worst of the worst.*

Top of the head: *There's no way I can forgive myself.*

Eyebrow: *There's no way others can forgive me.*

Side of the eye: *There's no way the Universe can forgive me.*

Under the eye: *I would like to forgive myself.*

Under the nose: *I know it would be good for me,*

Under the mouth: *But I just can't do it today.*

Collarbone: *All this shame and sadness I feel—*

Under arm: *I allow it all to be as it is.*

Top of the head: *And I do want to forgive myself.*

Eyebrow: *I want out of this prison of self-blame.*

Side of the eye: *I'm the only one keeping the door locked.*

Under the eye: *I give this stuck part of me my full attention.*

Under the nose: *This painfully stuck part of me—*

Under the mouth: *I give it all of my attention and all of my love.*

Collarbone: *This part of me that can't let go yet—*

Under arm: *I invite love to come into this part of my being.*

Top of the head: *I send love and understanding to this part of me*

Eyebrow: *That feels so scared and wounded and ashamed.*

Side of the eye: *Even if it's hard to let this love in,*

Under the eye: *I choose to let it in anyway*

Under the nose: *I love and accept this part of me just as it is,*

Under the mouth: *And I choose to trust that forgiveness will come*

Collarbone: *When I am ready and when the Universe is ready.*

Under arm: *In the meantime, I love myself exactly as I am in this moment.*

Take a nice deep breath. Check in with your initial distress level—is it higher, lower, or about the same? Keep repeating rounds of Tapping until you feel relief.

If you're struggling with an inability to forgive someone else, use this Tapping guide to jog those stuck parts loose.

Tapping Guide 11.2: "I Can't Forgive Others"

SETUP STATEMENT: *Even though I can't forgive [name] for what happened, I totally accept that this is how I feel.* (Say aloud one to three times.)

Top of the head: *I can't forgive [name].*

Eyebrow: *I completely refuse to forgive [name].*

Side of the eye: *I can't forgive [name] for what happened.*

Under the eye: *It's not fair that I should be the one to forgive.*

Under the nose: *What they did was so wrong.*

Under the mouth: *Why should I have to forgive?*

Collarbone: *If I forgive, it feels like what they did is okay.*

Under arm: *Forget that!*

Top of the head: *It feels unfair.*

Eyebrow: *I'm being chewed up internally*

Side of the eye: *By my lack of forgiveness.*

Under the eye: *I can't let go of my grudge.*

Under the nose: *All this resentment I feel—*

Under the mouth: *Poisoning my soul—*

Collarbone: *It's all their fault.*

Under arm: *If they hadn't done what they did, I would be fine.*

Top of the head: *Is that true?*

Eyebrow: *Is [name] in charge of my happiness?*

Side of the eye: *I've given away my power to [name].*

Under the eye: *I'm letting what [name] did run my life.*

Under the nose: *I don't want that anymore.*

Under the mouth: *I want to release this,*

Collarbone: *And it just feels stuck right now.*

Under arm: *I totally own and acknowledge this.*

Top of the head: *And as I own it,*

Eyebrow: *I become more open*

Side of the eye: *To how I can genuinely forgive this.*

Under the eye: *Maybe not all at once right now,*

Under the nose: *But just a little trickle,*

Under the mouth: *Getting stronger each day.*

Collarbone: *A little more forgiveness flows each day,*

Under arm: *As I love and acknowledge myself for how I feel.*

Take a nice deep breath. Check in with your initial distress level—is it higher, lower, or about the same? Keep repeating rounds of Tapping until you feel relief.

If you would like to forgive your body for its perceived shortcomings and learn to celebrate the beauty you are, join me in the following chapter, where I'll show you how to calm down that inner mean talk and let your light shine.

To tap along with audio recordings of this and other Tapping guides, visit www.marcellafriel.com/taptasteheal.

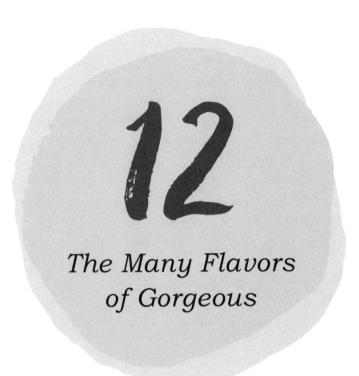

12

The Many Flavors of Gorgeous

I wake up every morning and decide to love my whole self.
—ISA, MODEL FOR #AerieREAL

WRITER'S BLOCK HAPPENS for a reason. It's no accident that I had dinner with my dear friend Jenny just as I was struggling with how to start this chapter. Jenny and I met up after her hairdresser appointment, and as we dined, she shared with me her deep ambivalence about the one-year process she'd undertaken to transition her hair color from bottle brown to natural gray.

"I don't know if I can go through with it," she confided. "I'm having a hard time getting away from the cultural imprinting about what it means to be attractive in the Western world right now. I feel an internal movement of wanting to let my hair go natural. It's a pain in the neck to keep coloring it and covering it, and it also feels energetically off to keep trying to cover something. There's a part of me that wants to take a stand and say, 'Ladies! We don't have to keep coloring our hair. We can be our natural gray and silver and still be attractive.' But when I actually see the gray, I realize that I can't escape my vanity. Plus, even though my partner says he's 100 percent fine with it, I wonder—if I don't look young and hot anymore, will he really still find me attractive?"

I sympathized with Jenny's dilemma, though not because I'm reticent about revealing my own graying locks. My hair struggle began at the opposite arc of the life cycle, in adolescence. Growing up in 1970s television-land, my role models for beauty were Barbie dolls and the *Brady Bunch* girls, wholesome blue-eyed teeny-boppers with corn-silk hair.

My appearance was a far fall from that pinnacle of perfection. The profuse frizzy brown hair that sprouted wildly from my crown chakra made me look like a cross between a young Bob Dylan and Eraserhead. My skin had the olive undertones of my Sicilian ancestors. I had a weird, ethnic first name. More than anything, I wanted desperately to be a Barbie-doll clone with a cute and perky nickname like *Skipper* or *Midge.*

At age twelve, I determined to take matters into my own hands and tame my wild Mediterranean mane once and for all. After spending a Saturday afternoon locked in the bathroom with chemical straightener and *SunIn* spray-on bleach, the result was a fried orange triangle of frizz akin to Gilda Radner's "Rosanne Rosannadanna" hairdo from the old *Saturday Night Live* days. I went to school the following Monday under a crimson pall of humiliation. The boys made obscene remarks that I cannot repeat to this day, implying that I was wearing a bush of pubic hair on my head.

Decades later, I stumbled across an article in *O* magazine written by a Puerto Rican woman who similarly struggled with the cultural messages of exclusion embedded in her hair. Reading and identifying with her story, I felt a surge of liberation in seeing a woman with hair like mine who played to her native beauty. After reading that article, I vowed never again to force my hair into something it was not. Thanks to that brave writer's example, I now wear my effusive locks with gratitude for my genetic inheritance.

The Monoculture of Appearance

We all feel grief and dismay over the loss of biodiversity on our Mother Earth. It wrenches our guts to read about the acres of pristine rainforest that are razed in a single day or to learn about yet another animal species on the verge of extinction. But what about the loss of human diversity? Activist and author Jerry Mander touches on this issue in his landmark book *In the Absence of the Sacred:*

> If there is one basic principle of environmentalism, it is that diversity is good. Beyond good, it is a bottom-line necessity for natural systems to survive. But the idea that communications technology, especially

television, can have a role in destroying diversity within the *human* realm is rarely noted.

By its ability to implant identical images into the minds of millions of people, television can homogenize perspectives, knowledge, tastes, and desires to make them resemble the tastes and interests of the people who transmit the imagery. In our world, the transmitters of the images are corporations whose ideal is technologically oriented, commodity oriented, materialistic, and hostile to nature.[1]

The term *monoculture* typically refers to the industrial custom of sowing genetically identical plants across vast acres of land. Over time, this depletes soil, increases dependence on chemical inputs, and threatens the health of the plants themselves. And just as crop monoculture threatens the natural diversity of our food choices, the narrow definition of beauty as propagated by the fashion industry is squeezing cultural, racial, and body-size diversity into a monoculture of appearance, especially among girls and women. Millions of us have identical images implanted in our minds of what our bodies are supposed to look like. If we're not white, young, size triple 0, and seven feet tall, we simply do not qualify as attractive, much less beautiful. For the 98 percent of us who don't look like fashion models, the toxic harvest of the beauty monoculture is a contempt of our bodies that is seared into our soul like a cattle brand.

According to Taryn Brumfitt, creator of the documentary film *Embrace,* seven out of ten women on this planet hate their bodies. In the United States, 53 percent of all thirteen-year-old girls are unhappy with their appearance; by age seventeen, that figure balloons to 78 percent.[2] The word girls and women most commonly use to describe their bodies is *disgusting.*[3]

The average woman in the United States stands 5′4″ tall and weighs 140 pounds. The average model in the United States is 5′11″ and weighs 117 pounds. Sixty-nine percent of girls in one study reported that magazine models influence their ideal of the perfect body shape. Forty-seven percent of those girls reported wanting to lose weight, but only 29 percent actually were overweight. Girls who already felt dissatisfaction with their bodies showed more dieting, anxiety, and bulimic symptoms after prolonged exposure to fashion and advertising images in magazines aimed at teen girls.

The average US woman sees about five hundred advertisements per day. Half of the ads and television commercials directed at female viewers use physical attractiveness to promote products. By the time a girl is seventeen, she has received over a quarter million such messages through the media. This constant exposure drives girls and women to loathe their bodies, measure their self-worth by their physical appearance, and dread growing older, which is perceived as tantamount to becoming unattractive.[4]

Some researchers believe that advertisers purposely normalize unrealistically thin bodies in order to create an unattainable desire that will drive product consumption. Paul Hamburg, assistant professor of psychiatry at Harvard Medical School, writes, "The media markets desire. And by reproducing ideals that are absurdly out of line with what real bodies really look like, the media perpetuates a market for frustration and disappointment. Its customers will never disappear."[5]

The Shame That's Not Ours

What do you say to yourself when you see your own image in the mirror?

- "Look at my gut!"
- "I look disgusting!"
- "I feel like such a pig!"
- "My thighs are enormous!"
- "I've got Fat Cow Disease!"
- "I look like a beached whale!"

You probably wouldn't dream of saying such harmful words to your best friend, but you don't think twice about saying these things to yourself. Whether you say them aloud or not, the body shaming you internalize and inflict on yourself keeps you stuck in your past, undermines your confidence, demolishes your self-trust, and creates metabolic conditions that make weight loss total hell.

Brené Brown, a therapist and researcher who specializes in shame and vulnerability, defines *shame* as "the intensely painful feeling of believing that we are flawed and therefore unworthy of love, belonging, and connection."[6] Whereas *guilt* is the recognition of having made a mistake, Brown says that *shame* spawns the belief that we are the mistake. "Guilt says, 'I did something bad'; shame says, 'I am bad.'"

Shame feeds on secrecy and silence just as yeast feeds on sugar. So when we expose our unspoken shame to the light of day, we discover something surprising: even though we feel it so personally, *shame is not really ours*. None of us emerges *ex utero* feeling shame. In the course of our lives, we pick up shame like a sticky toxic goo in response to our perceived failure to meet expectations that someone, somewhere, decided we should meet. There's family-of-origin shame, cultural shame, racial shame, gender shame, sexuality shame, economic shame, educational shame, marital-status shame, body-size shame—the list goes on and on.

When I challenged my client Priya, who immigrated to the United States from India, to consider that she might be more addicted to her chronic stress than to her food choices, she gasped in shock. Then, after a moment of introspection, she said, "There could be some wisdom to what you say, Marcella. If I think about being addicted to stress, I see that I am constantly go-go-going, trying to achieve, because I did not become a doctor or an engineer, like a good Indian."

Think for a moment about where you feel vulnerable to shame. (You might want to place one or both hands on your heart as you do this.) Perhaps you feel shame about your parenting skills, your body size, or your financial predicament. As best you can, feel that shame without judging yourself.

Then take a deeper look. Whose shame is it *really?* Is this shame intrinsic to who you are? Or is it the result of messages that you picked up along the way about how someone—whether an individual, a tribe, or a society—believes you *should* be? (If the shame feels especially strong, go ahead and jump to the Shame Detox Ritual that follows; otherwise, hang in there with me while I unpack this issue a little further.)

The good news about shame is that if it's learned, it can be unlearned. And Tapping is a great tool for quickly detoxifying our inherited legacy of shame, wherever it came from. When tapping, there often comes a moment when the brain's limbic system spontaneously releases the presenting distress. This happened for me one day while tapping on my own shame. I realized that anything I felt ashamed of—growing up in poverty, being the daughter of a jailbird father and a mentally ill mother, having a checkered and picaresque relationship history—I could just as easily feel proud of and grateful for.

When I allowed myself to wade through the swampland of my shame, to touch and love and tap on the lonely parts of me that believed that my value on this earth was determined by the circumstances of my birth or that my worth as a woman was only in relation to a man, I was able to pry the story lines loose from the reality. Rather than torturing myself with the beliefs that I shouldn't have grown up poor or that I should have gotten married or that I shouldn't have slept with so many people, I began to see, as Byron Katie says, "It should have happened this way because it did happen this way.… No one can give you free-dom but you."[7]

I began flipping my shameful beliefs on their head. What can I be proud of about these circumstances? I'm proud that my poor background motivated me to become financially self-supporting. I'm proud of what I learned from and about my many lovers and what I learned from and about myself. Far from being shame-ful, my history began to reveal the gold amid the dross—the complex, poignant, vulnerable, and beautiful phoenix of Marcella rose from her own ashes: pristine, perfect, flawless. Yes, it certainly should have happened this way. I wouldn't trade a moment of it for anything else.

Shame Detox Ritual

If you would like to release the shame that has bound you, this is a great ritual to do alone, with a friend, or in the presence of someone who genuinely supports you. Set aside about thirty minutes for this ritual. You'll need several scraps of paper, a pen, a candle, a cauldron (a vessel for burning the paper), and a quiet place free from interruption.

> Begin by lighting the candle and sitting for a few minutes in silence, until your everyday awareness has shifted into a more settled space.
>
> On each scrap of paper, write: "I now release my shame over _____." Write each cause of shame on a separate scrap of paper.
>
> When you have them all written down, read them aloud, one by one. After you read each one, crumple up that piece of paper and throw it into the cauldron.
>
> Place one or both hands on your heart and contemplate deeply what you are releasing. Are you truly ready to release your identification with this shame as who you are?
>
> When you're ready, burn the paper.
>
> After you're complete, body-brush yourself—or invite your witness to body-brush you. Starting at the top of your head, brush your body with your hands on all sides, using downward strokes, as if you're brushing something off of you or away from you. (If you're doing the ritual with a friend, you can take turns body-brushing each other.) You might also want to vocalize your release of the shame (laugh, yell, howl, sing) during the body brushing.

When the body brushing is complete, sit again in silence, with your hands on your heart, and let your awareness rest in the space of the released shame.

Blow out the candle, and you're done.

Buh-bye, shame.

Perfect Is Predictable—Be Amazing Instead

For women, shame frequently shows up through its malevolent twin, *perfectionism:* the trap of unattainable, conflicting expectations we internalize and perpetuate about who we believe we are supposed to be. Perfectionism tells us to be nice, be thin, be modest, have it all together, always take care of others before yourself, and never allow anyone to see your needs or vulnerability. Anything less is simply unacceptable. "When perfectionism is driving," says Brené Brown, "shame is riding shotgun. And fear is the back-seat driver. [Perfectionism] says: 'If I look perfect, live perfect, or work perfect, I can avoid or minimize criticism, blame, and ridicule.'"[8]

If you grew up in an intensely shaming environment, you might well have a terrified little one inside you who decided that being perfect was the best way to deflect the pain of the shame. That's an incredibly wise stance for a child who has no other protection mechanisms available. But if you, as an adult, take a deeper look at perfectionism, you might see that it's not only impossible—it's also ultimately undesirable.

Trying to be perfect ensures you will always strive toward your desired goal but never get to a point that satisfies you enough to feel that you've actually arrived.[9] Every action you take becomes grimly laden with the ponderous pressure to do it perfectly, or else it has no value at all.

When you do reach your goal—say, you attain your ideal body weight—your inner mean voice will say, "yes, but …" and tell you that it could have been better, or you could do more, or it doesn't really count, because of such-and-such. Perfectionism rubs your nose in every perceived mistake, ensuring that you take no joy in your accomplishment. No matter how perfect you already are, perfectionism convinces you that it—and you—are never enough.

Plus, being perfect is … well, boring. There's no heartbeat inside of perfectionism, no crack where the light shines out or in, no humanity that others can relate to. Perfectionism is a hyperbaric chamber of isolation, which explains why so many people who do, in fact, reach their ideal body weight often feel miserable when it's achieved in this way. While perfectionism can protect you from ridicule, it also prevents you from experiencing life-affirming intimacy with yourself and others.

When we reclaim our dignity from the stories we tell ourselves about what's hopelessly wrong with us, when we drop our shoulds and shouldn'ts down the "should hole" and really cut ourselves free, we get to enjoy ourselves as the terrific people we truly are, and we get to revel in the freedom that comes from being *amazing* instead of being *perfect*.

On Her Own Terms

It's high time that we collectively disabuse ourselves of the idea that body thinness is the only way to achieve beauty, health, happiness, success, fulfillment, and self-esteem. Fortunately, the tide is turning in this direction, with legions of heroines leading the way.

Tess Holliday is a stunningly gorgeous size-22 model who did not wait for the fashion industry to give her the green light before claiming and proclaiming the beauty she is. Among the myriad tattoos that festoon her generous arms are images of country-music icon Dolly Parton, sex-positive actress Mae West, legendary drag queen Divine, and *Sesame Street*'s Miss Piggy. Of the latter, Holliday says, "Miss Piggy's there because she's awesome. She's glamorous and sassy and funny, like me."[10] Tess's looks are on her own terms. By challenging the mainstream fashion industry's tyrannically impossible standards, she is creating a new paradigm of authentic feminine body confidence and paving the way for others to follow in her footsteps.

In January 2014, the clothing company American Eagle announced that it would discontinue using digitally retouched images of supermodels and launched the #AerieREAL campaign (#aeriereal), aimed at young women ages fifteen to twenty-four and featuring models of various colors, shapes, sizes, and physical abilities, replete with tattoos, braces, shaved heads, skin variations, and beauty marks. The Aerie lingerie line features bras and bralettes for girls sizes 30A to 40DDD, worn by models with similar body types. Aerie is also the first national retailer to sponsor the American Eating Disorders Association and to raise funds for educational initiatives for eating disorders.[11]

Redbook magazine has likewise jumped on the body-love train by featuring curvy models in its annual swimwear issue, released each June. As Meredith

Rollins, *Redbook*'s editor, explains, "We make sure to shoot [the issue] with a woman who has gorgeous curves, because that's true for most of our readers, it's true for women in general, and to celebrate a gorgeous, healthy, curvy body. The pictures are very joyful, which I think is important."[12]

After numerous futile attempts to alligator-wrestle her body into its prepubescent size, my client Georgia, then twenty-four years old, decided to jettison the body shame and celebrate her present-time appearance. She described to me how good it felt finally to purchase her first plus-sized outfit and work with her body rather than against it. In an Instagram photo rocking her sassy new clothes, she posted, "Our bodies change and respond to all the elements of our lives. It can be incredibly frustrating—and then there are moments of liberation—like this one brought on by this adorable plaid plus-size set. My body will continue to change as I am ever changing, and it's my job to try and respect myself in all stages. And for now, accepting the fact that I'm a more curvy gal than I've ever been, I aim to rock it."

Love Your Mother, Love Yourself

If you still find it hard to imagine that there could be anything beautiful about your appearance, take a wide-lens view of the natural world around you. Mother Nature always expresses her beauty in diversity. She hasn't given us just one type of beautiful flower. Think of the delicacy of a shrinking violet, the captivating complexity of a peony, the blazing cheerfulness of a sunflower, the allure of a tiger lily, the flamboyance of a bird-of-paradise. Can you really say one is more beautiful than the other? Can you really think that all of them should imitate a store-bought rose? Genuine beauty always is kaleidoscopic in nature—it continually shape-shifts, revealing a new facet with each change.

Our bodies are inseparable from Mother Nature's design, and so to hate our bodies is to hate our mother. We would never litter or shave off the top of a mountain; we wouldn't dump toxins into our backyard creek or mow down an old-growth forest. It's time, then, to stop polluting our precious bodies with toxic thoughts of "not good enough" and to reclaim our reverence for them as miraculous offspring of our precious mother.

As you know by now, in the Tapping world we use affirmations of self-love, such as, "I deeply love and accept myself exactly as I am," to dissipate our emotional distress. The first time I had to say these words aloud to another person, I thought it was the most hokey, schmaltzy, new-agey thing I could ever imagine saying. The EFT practitioner I worked with at the time encouraged me to say it anyway—"fake it till you make it"—and I'm so glad she did. After saying that phrase thousands, perhaps tens of thousands of times, the schmaltz has given way to a self-love I can own.

In our culture, it's far, far more customary and acceptable to hate ourselves than it is to love ourselves. Within society at large, within our communities, and within our families of origin, we receive subtle and not-so-subtle admonitions against holding ourselves too much in a positive regard, lest we become narcissistic. But is that what will happen?

Narcissism has its roots in the Greek myth of Narcissus, a young man who fell in love with his own reflection in a pond and then killed himself when he realized the image could never become the man of his dreams. The myth is referenced as a cautionary tale: Don't be too prideful about your appearance. Something terrible will happen if you are.

I looked up the story. Turns out Narcissus was a real jerk. His godlike appearance notwithstanding, Narcissus heaped scorn and contempt on those who were charmed by his good looks.[13] He rejected Echo, a nymph who had fallen in love with him, by mimicking her every word until she faded away, leaving nothing behind but the sound of her voice. Narcissus spurned many lovers, among them a fellow named Ameinias, who committed suicide imploring the goddess Nemesis to curse Narcissus for his heartlessness.[14] Narcissus wasn't a jerk because he fell in love with himself. He was—well, *narcissistic*—way before he met his fate. Yet this story is not told as an encouragement to be kind to others. It's told as an admonition to shine our light at low wattage, if at all.

True self-love is a far cry from pathological self-centeredness. Relationship doyenne Tracy McMillan, in her TEDx talk "The Person You Really Need to Marry," puts it this way:

> You don't say to yourself, "When you lose ten pounds, then I'll love you." … Maybe you don't own a home … you didn't get the career you wanted … you fight with your mom or watch too much reality TV. Whatever it is, it doesn't matter anymore. Because when you marry yourself, you agree to stay with *you* no matter what.
>
> What I learned in [the ending of] my third marriage was how to sit at my own bedside and how to hold my own hand, and how to nurse myself and comfort myself. And what I learned from that is, I am a person I can count on.

When you love yourself fully, you can love other people right where they are, for who they are, in the same way you're already loving yourself. And of course, this is what the world needs more of.[15]

"Hello Beautiful"

If the thought of self-love still makes you queasy, take baby steps toward it, one day at a time—of self-appreciation, self-understanding, and self-kindness. Facials and pedicures are nice, but they're not the same as a rock-solid commitment to yourself, as you are in this moment, that says, "I am with you no matter what."

Try this, and see what happens. Every day—after, say, washing your face before bed—look deeply at your face in the mirror. Look all the way in to the pupils of your eyes—the only part of your body that has not changed since the day you were born. As you look, say aloud to yourself, "Hello Beautiful." Say it again. One more time. Let it resonate. Say it to yourself as you would have a loved one say it to you. Say it repeatedly, until it sinks in, and you realize and embody its truth.

What Might Be Possible

Take a breath for a moment and consider: What might open up in your life if you could drop the shame and live from your intrinsic beauty and worthiness, whatever your shape or size? What if you could befriend your body and allow it to guide you to the foods that satisfy your genuine hunger? What if you could find safety and peace in stopping when you are contentedly full? What if you stopped punishing yourself with exercise regimens that you don't do anyway, and instead allowed your body to do what it loves—gardening, dancing, gentle yoga, rolling around on the floor, taking easy hikes in the hills, cuddling with your beloved?

Most important, what if you could turn away from the brutally perfectionistic standards of how the fashion industry says you should look and give your body unconditional love and acceptance as it is? What if, when the body-shaming inner talk arose, you could slow down, step back, place your hands on your heart, take three deep, conscious breaths, and say, "Some deeper part of me is calling out for love, and my job right now is to become inquisitive and listen"? How might our society and our planet heal if we could reclaim ourselves in this way?

Let's Do Some Tapping

Whatever the roots of your body shame, use this Tapping guide to shift into deep appreciation and gratitude for the miracle that is your body.

Before we begin tapping, I'm going to ask you to do something that might be uncomfortable: Strip down as far as you feel comfortable and stand in front of a full-length mirror, if you have one. Tune in to where you feel the shame. What parts of your body trigger shame for you? And how intense does that shame feel, on a scale of 1 to 10, with 10 being the most intense? Once you have all that dialed in, begin.

Tapping Guide 12.1: "I Feel Ashamed of My Body"

SETUP STATEMENT: *Even though I feel all this shame about my body, I choose to love myself as best I can right now.* (Say aloud one to three times.)

Top of the head: *All this body shame I feel—*

Eyebrow: *It's really horrible.*

Side of the eye: *All this body shame that I carry—*

Under the eye: *I feel so deeply ashamed of my body.*

Under the nose: *This painful, intense, stuck feeling—*

Under the mouth: *It feels like a prison and a trap.*

Collarbone: *I can't imagine how I can ever get free of it.*

Under arm: *This body shame is so deep.*

Top of the head: *I've been carrying this shame so long.*

Eyebrow: *It feels like who I am.*

Side of the eye: *This mean inner voice*

Under the eye: *That says* [insert mean, shaming self-talk here]—

Under the nose: *That voice wants to keep me stuck and ashamed.*

Under the mouth: *I know I'm stuck here,*

Collarbone: *But I don't want to stay stuck here.*

Under arm: *I really want to move past this.*

Top of the head: *I am open to shifting this.*

Eyebrow: *I really want to set myself free—*

Side of the eye: *Release this awful shame—*

Under the eye: *But I have no idea how to do that.*

Under the nose: *Whose shame is this, anyway?*

Under the mouth: *Wherever I got these beliefs*

Collarbone: *That say* [insert mean, shaming self-talk here]—

Under arm: *What if I could let them go?*

Top of the head: *I want to stop believing this shame.*

Eyebrow: *It really never was mine.*

Side of the eye: *Wherever this shame came from,*

Under the eye: *I'm sending it back with a thousandfold increase in consciousness.*

Under the nose: *Whoever passed this shame on to me—*

Under the mouth: *May you be healed.*

Collarbone: *May I be healed.*

Under arm: *Let's get out of the shadows together.*

Take a nice deep breath. Check in with your initial distress level—is it higher, lower, or about the same? Keep repeating rounds of Tapping until you feel relief.

Before you tap along with this Tapping guide, contemplate and complete the following sentences:

- "I can't be beautiful as I am because _____."

- "I would love to shine my true beauty, but _____."

Keep these two sentences in mind as you tap. Feel free to insert that language into this Tapping guide.

Tapping Guide 12.2: "If I'm Not Thin, I'm Not Beautiful"

SETUP STATEMENT: *Even though I feel that I have to be thin to be beautiful, and some part of me knows this isn't true, while another part of me can't help feeling that way, I deeply love myself exactly where I'm at.* (Say aloud one to three times.)

Top of the head: *I have to be thin to be beautiful.*

Eyebrow: *I have to be thin.*

Side of the eye: *Otherwise I'm just not attractive.*

Under the eye: *How can someone like me be beautiful?*

Under the nose: *I don't want to feel this way.*

Under the mouth: *I want to love my body as it is*

Collarbone: *And see my real beauty,*

Under arm: *But I'm just not there yet.*

Top of the head: *I have to be thin to be beautiful.*

Eyebrow: *I have to have a perfect body—*

Side of the eye: *Whatever that means—*

Under the eye: *In order to be beautiful.*

Under the nose: *What makes me not beautiful as I am?*

Under the mouth: *I'm picking my body apart,*

Collarbone: *Giving myself such a hard time—*

Under arm: *All this judgment and cruelty toward myself.*

Top of the head: *It doesn't help me look better or feel better.*

Eyebrow: *Criticizing my body will not make me beautiful.*

Side of the eye: *I want to stop being so mean to myself.*

Under the eye: *I want to love myself as I am.*

Under the nose: *Is that okay?*

Under the mouth: *Can I give myself permission?*

Collarbone: *What if I could let go of torturing myself,*

Under arm: *And let myself shine just as I am?*

Top of the head: *I choose to shine my light.*

Eyebrow: *Who says I have to be thin, anyway?*

Side of the eye: *Perhaps I can be beautiful as I am—*

Under the eye: *Relaxing and letting myself shine,*

Under the nose: *Letting go of all the torture,*

Under the mouth: *Shining my sweet gorgeous light,*

Collarbone: *Celebrating the beauty I am.*

Under arm: *I choose to begin right in this moment.*

Take a nice deep breath. Check in with your initial distress level—is it higher, lower, or about the same? Keep repeating rounds of Tapping until you feel relief.

In the next chapter, let me share with you the most profound and joyous ecological tool available to heal your body, your life, and Mother Earth herself.

To tap along with audio recordings of this and other Tapping guides, visit www .marcellafriel.com/taptasteheal.

13

Your Life Is the Supreme Meal

Zen masters call a life that is lived fully, with nothing held back, "the supreme meal." And a person who lives such a life—a person who knows how to plan, cook, appreciate, serve, and offer the supreme meal of life—is called a Zen cook.

—BERNIE GLASSMAN, ROSHI

IN MODERN LIFE, our collective drug of choice is "more, better, cheaper, quicker." In our frenzy to shield ourselves against any sharp edges of reality Mother Earth might send our way, we take refuge in efficiency, convenience, and speed at the expense of process, appreciation, and quality. We consume and toss not just food but entertainment, relationships, spirituality, perhaps even our own lives.

In a world where pleasure is commodified, joy is marketed, and eating is just a matter of shoveling in calories so we can get to the next thing on our list, our lives have degenerated into mere survival, rushing from one thing to another in an epidemic of "hurry sickness" that depletes our energy and ransacks Mother Earth's natural generosity.

The epitome of this barbarianism is the drive-through meal. We don't have to take time to get out of the car, sit at a table, be served, eat properly, and clean up, as our ancestors have done for centuries before us. We don't have to be present to the food, to the hands that prepared it, to our bodies as we ingest it. When we're done, we throw uneaten remains into the trash, along with the polymer packaging that will clog Mother Earth's belly for the next half-million years. Everything is a means to an end that never arrives, until, one day, our body—and our planet— presents the bill.

Bottomless Bowls

Recently I had lunch with a friend; I ordered a Caesar salad with chicken. What arrived at the table was a mountain of romaine lettuce large enough to rival the fourteen-thousand-foot peaks in my Colorado backyard. This was not one, but at least six full portions of salad, intended for one person. I shrugged, sighed, ate a few forkfuls, and pushed the rest away. And no, I didn't take a doggie bag of soggy lettuce home to sit in my fridge before I threw it out.

Leaving the restaurant, I sadly recalled meditation master Chögyam Trungpa's words in his book *Shambhala: The Sacred Path of the Warrior:* "When people go to restaurants, often they are served giant platefuls of food, more than they can eat, to satisfy the giant desire of their minds. Their minds are stuffed just by the visual appearance of their giant steaks, their full plates."[1]

In our modern industrial food culture, we face a dilemma that our hunter-gatherer ancestors would have never imagined possible: the overabundance of food in supermarkets and the supersized portions at restaurants present us with more than we can possibly eat. In the United States and Canada, we throw out about 40 percent of the food on our plates (compared to 4 percent in sub-Saharan Africa). Globally, according to the United Nations Food and Agriculture Organization, one out of three pounds of all food prepared for consumption on this planet is wasted.[2] This global squander sends 3.3 billion tons of carbon into the atmosphere and consumes about seven hundred square miles of water—an amount three times the size of Lake Geneva in Switzerland.

"Food waste—it's kind of the tip of the iceberg," says Jason Clay, a senior vice-president in charge of food policy at the World Wildlife Fund.[3] And according to global climate activist Lynne Twist, we're consuming planetary resources—soil and water specifically—50 percent faster than they can replenish themselves.[4] Given these dire facts, and given the increasing temperatures and bizarre weather patterns we are now all experiencing, it's absolutely time for us—right now, starting today—to make sure that the food we buy we will, in fact, eat.

It's also high time to prevail upon the eateries we patronize to right-size their serving portions. Since the 1990s, portion sizes have doubled or tripled, a key factor contributing not only to global environmental devastation but also to the physical and emotional anguish of those who suffer from chronic, compulsive overeating and its myriad consequences. If I had that lunch with my friend to do again, I would have mentioned to my food server that the salad was way too big. Most retailers know that if five customers ask for something, it's time to make a change. Let's all be among those five and speak up.[5]

In 2005, researchers at Cornell University's Food Lab had fifty-four subjects eat soup.[6] Half were served soup in normal bowls with normal portion sizes. The other half were served from a bowl that was imperceptibly, incrementally refilled through a tube beneath the table. The subjects who unknowingly ate from the self-refilling bowls consumed an average of 73 percent more soup without perceiving themselves as eating more or being more full than their counterparts. When we eat from seemingly bottomless bowls of food, several things happen:

- *We eat from our eyes, not from our bellies.* We let the amount of food on the plate, rather than our body, tell us how much we should eat. Our body's *satiety cues*—the messages between brain and belly that say that we have had enough—go haywire. We lose our sense of where full ends and overstuffed begins.

- *We feel guilty.* We've all heard the admonition, "Eat your food! There are children starving in the world!" If we have any social conscience at all, we feel the pain of inequitable food access and distribution around the planet. But overstuffing ourselves does not alleviate the hunger of others. As Frances Moore Lappé said in her classic book *Diet for a Small Planet,* hunger is not caused by lack of food but by lack of democracy.[7] Eating more food than our bodies can handle is not the antidote to global starvation.

- *We get fatter.* Marion Nestle, a professor of nutrition, food studies, and public health at New York University, positively correlates obesity rates with supersized food portions: "The larger portion business started at exactly the same time that obesity rates started to go up. … Muffins used to be one or two ounces; now they're six or seven or eight. … When I was a kid, bagels were the size of what are now called mini-bagels. And you never used to go into a restaurant and be presented with a bowl of pasta that would feed six people."[8]

Perhaps the most tragic and pervasive consequence of our perpetual food surplus is that we don't appreciate the food we have; we regard eating as more of a chore than a pleasure. If, as food journalist Michael Pollan says, "The banquet is in the first bite,"[9] there's no point in savoring our excessive fare if none of it is precious to us. "In the developed world, food is more abundant, but it costs much less," says Rosa Rolle, an expert on food and waste at the UN Food and Agriculture Organization, "but people don't value food for what it represents."[10]

When society functions strictly on the basis of efficiency, everyone loses (except those who stand to profit from it, but even that's only a short-term gain). And in a food system designed for us simply to stuff calories into our bodies, we are set up to become disembodied as we eat. Why bother to feed ourselves well or eat mindfully if the whole function of food is simply to overfill our guts? If the only purpose of food is to provide nutrition, why bother looking for the best meat, the best butter, the best vegetables? And if, indeed, you are what you eat, do you really want to be cheap, fast, and easy? And if not, what is the antidote?

The Deep Ecology of Gratitude

The more I look at appreciation and gratitude, the more I see them as the most ecological tools we have to heal not only our bodies but the entire planet. Appreciation and gratitude have a double-helix relationship—they augment each other. We can be grateful, for example, for the food we have in our lives, but when we slow down to *appreciate* the food—to notice the presentation, the aromas, the nutrition, the preparation, and the flavor—we amplify our gratitude by recognizing the myriad gifts good food brings us every day. Conversely, when we take time to consider *why* we're grateful, we're led inevitably to appreciate *what* we're grateful for.

Before we get into any more mushy-gushy stuff about how wonderful these qualities are to cultivate, let's look at them for a moment through their shadow side. *Regret* and *resentment*—the opposites of gratitude and appreciation—are easy, cheap, and everywhere, like junk food. Just as we throw away the drive-through packaging without a second thought, the energy of *regret* and *resentment* prompt us to see our lives only as waste to be discarded. "I'm a failure." "I should have done it by now." "What's the use?" "It's too late for me." "I'm not worth it." "It's not worth it." "Things will never get any better." "If only [fill in the blank] hadn't happened, my life would be fine."

Instead of seeing the potential value in our experience, whether pleasurable or painful, we just want to get out of the pain, throw our experience away, get rid of it. We don't care where it goes, as long as it's not in our backyard. This is the same energy that litters highways, dumps poison into rivers, and causes us to trash and punish ourselves for what we see as our shortcomings.

If resentment is a form of energetic debt, as I described in chapter 11, then appreciation and gratitude are the means by which we increase our spiritual wealth portfolio and prepare the supreme meal that is our life.

As a culture, we typically sequester our gratitude for Thanksgiving (which, curiously enough, is our national high holy day of overeating). We're taught that gratitude means sitting around a table that's overfull with food and giving thanks in the manner of a child petitioning Santa Claus: "Thank you, God, for this; Thank you, God, for that." It's easy to be grateful when you have a feast before you. But what about when your bowl is empty? How can we find gratitude and appreciation for something as painful as our food and body-love struggles?

In his early Buddhist teachings, Chögyam Trungpa wrote of "the manure of experience and the field of *bodhi* (or wakefulness)":[11]

> Unskilled farmers throw out their rubbish and buy manure from other farmers; but skilled farmers collect their manure, in spite of the bad smell and the unclean work, and spread it on their land, and out of this they grow their crops.
>
> If a person is skilled enough and patient enough to sift through his rubbish and study it thoroughly, he will … develop a positive outlook and create great wealth.

When you seek to effect change of any kind from a place of resentment, you are throwing away your rubbish and looking outside yourself to see if some other manure is better than what you already have. You're adding more pollution to the problem. The path of appreciation, by contrast, teaches us how to become a skilled farmer of our own soul: how to use the manure of our experience to fertilize the soil that grows our crops, which we then use to prepare the supreme meal of our precious life. In the words of Bernie Glassman, coauthor of *Instructions to the Cook: A Zen Master's Lessons in Living a Life That Matters,* "The supreme meal—your own life—is the greatest gift you can receive and the greatest offering you can make."[12]

How do we prepare such a meal? We begin with giving up our preferences for one kind of experience over another. We stop craving happiness and rejecting sadness and instead recognize, with an equal eye, that both have their merits and their drawbacks. We stop fighting ourselves and acknowledge what is. In the Zen cook's language, we work with the ingredients in our pantry. Perhaps we open the cupboard, and all we see is sorrow, struggle, and loss. We can appreciate those bitter, pungent, and astringent flavors as wakeful contrasts to our incessant craving for sweetness, which lulls us to sleep and makes us allergic to discomfort and growth.

In the practice of Tapping, we say, "Even though I have this problem, I deeply and completely love and accept myself." In the view of Tapping, self-love, self-appreciation, and self-acceptance are the antidotes to every stressful situation we can experience. Like a high-quality salt, appreciation harmonizes all the flavors of our life and brings out their most beneficial nutrients.

As our Tapping practice helps us grow into unconditional self-acceptance, we begin to see our struggles in a very different way. They shape-shift from a source of self-hatred to a rich, ripe, smelly, fertile gateway to wisdom and compassion. As we dowse the wreckage of our traumas to reveal the gifts, blessings, and lessons within them, we come to appreciate that sometimes the worst things that we can experience are the greatest blessings in disguise. Had we thrown out our rubbish and bought our manure elsewhere, we would have squandered the wealth right in our own garden.

When our life becomes the supreme meal, we clean up. We appreciate ourselves enough not to gossip about our coworker; we appreciate ourselves enough to get to bed at a reasonable hour, so we can get up earlier and make a good breakfast; we appreciate ourselves enough to take the thirty-minute walk we've been promising ourselves; we appreciate ourselves enough to naturally abstain from that which does not serve us and to cultivate that which does. We realize, ultimately, that nothing—*nothing*—is ever out of place. Our entire journey becomes a sacred unity and thus worthy of our deepest reverence and gratitude.

Cultivating Food Peace and Body Love

There are many reasons why gratitude and appreciation are the key ingredients to your supreme meal:

> *Gratitude improves physical health.* Negative emotions such as resentment and anger trigger the body's inflammatory and stress responses, which, in

turn, trigger food cravings and cause the body to hold on to excess weight. Gratitude, by contrast, cools the heat and inspires you to stretch yourself beyond these small-minded emotions and notch up your self-care.

- *Gratitude improves sleep.* If you spend fifteen minutes at night journaling about what you're grateful for from the day, chances are excellent your sleep will improve. And regular, restful sleep is one of the most important components of sustained and successful weight loss and mental well-being.

- *Gratitude improves self-esteem.* You stop comparing your insides to others' outsides and coming up better than or less than. Gratitude helps you find your right-sized place in your world, which can then translate into finding your right-sized physique.

- *Gratitude fosters resilience and reduces trauma.* People who regularly express and experience appreciation have fewer PTSD symptoms and more resilience during stressful circumstances, which keeps every metabolic system in the body on even keel.

- *Gratitude magnetizes resources.* As the saying goes, "You catch more bees with honey than you do with vinegar." Gratitude delightfully sends friends, opportunities, money, and other auspicious conditions your way when you least expect them and most need them.

A Path to the Source

Perhaps the greatest benefit of practicing gratitude and appreciation is that they plug us into an ever-renewable bank of energy, a cup that always overflows and never runs dry. In twelve-step lingo, that energy is called "the God of Your Understanding," which goes by many names:

- Allah
- The Angels
- Atman
- Buddha Nature
- The Divine Mother
- God

- 🌿 The Goddess
- 🌿 Great Spirit
- 🌿 HaShem
- 🌿 Higher Power
- 🌿 The Infinite
- 🌿 Source Energy
- 🌿 Spirit
- 🌿 Universal Love
- 🌿 The Unmanifest Absolute

Cultivating a consistent, conscious connection with this unseen animating force is, in my humble opinion, the single most powerful tool we have for finding hope in the rubble of despair, order in the wreckage of chaos, a way in the midst of no way. As Amma, the guru known for her life-changing hugs, likes to say, "Take one step toward God, and God takes one hundred steps toward you."

Meal Prayers and Blessings

What better way, then, to heal our chronic afflictions with food than to invite that source energy, the God of Our Understanding, to join us at the dinner table? There is, ultimately, no better way to overcome unhealthy food behaviors than to practice sincere, mindful appreciation for your food in the form of meal prayers and blessings.

Addiction expert Gabor Maté points out that the ceremonial use of a substance is the direct opposite of the addictive use. Whereas food addictions reinforce our alienation in a hostile world, food rituals elevate our consciousness and celebrate our connection to a larger, benevolent universe. They also, according to chef and nutritionist Rebecca Katz, downshift our nervous system out of fight-or-flight mode and into a parasympathetic state, which makes our food easier to digest.

My favorite mealtime prayer is simply putting my hands on my heart, closing my eyes, and taking three deep, conscious breaths before I eat. Much like bowing before entering a meditation hall, such a gesture creates an energetic transition from everyday speed into sacred space. Spiritual traditions from every culture have beautiful meal prayers you can draw from if you need training wheels for this practice. You can also borrow this prayer I wrote for the first mindful-eating class I ever taught:

> In this meal, the five elements offer themselves for my nourishment.
> To the sun that provides light, warmth, and growth,
> to the rain that replenishes and makes whole,
> to the father wind that scatters the sacred seed,
> to the mother earth that bears the seed in her fertile womb,
> and to the space that gives birth to the dance of the elements,
> I, your youngest daughter, offer thanks and praise.
> On behalf of all sentient beings, I gratefully receive and enjoy this meal. Amen.

You're also welcome to use the prayer my client Pam wrote. (As she noted, "You can't shovel crap into your mouth after saying this!"): "Before I was able to nourish myself, I was provided nourishment with great love and care. May I always love myself enough to give my body this gift of health and compassion. May I always respect the earth that provided this meal, and the hands that worked so hard to raise, grow, and shape the ingredients into the meal I am about to eat."

I do encourage you, whenever you are ready, to write your own meal prayer. Say it at least once a day and see how it changes your relationship with your food.

Simple Tools for Appreciative Eating

Once you have served the supreme meal, how do you eat it? Here are some tools for appreciative eating that I've cobbled together from various spiritual traditions. These guidelines bring peaceful delight to the table and have helped me and my clients reclaim sanity, choice, and dignity in our eating habits while cultivating love of our food and ourselves.

Eat food prepared by loving hands in a loving way.

This rule is simple but not always easy. If you're eating processed food, do you know whose hands—if anyone's—prepared it? If you're chronically dining on packaged foods or takeout, chances are human hands barely even touched what you eat. What kind of nourishment can you draw from such "food"—or rather, "foodlike products"—that are made by production machinery? Treat yourself to genuine nourishment. Eat at a local mom-and-pop restaurant instead of going to a fast-food joint. Visit a farmers' market, join a CSA (community-supported agriculture) group, learn to cook a few simple things on your own, or ask friends and family to cook for you.

Pause before you eat.

Stop. Close your eyes. If it's comfortable to do so, place your hands on your heart and take three deep, conscious breaths. If not, affirm your intention, through some sort of prayer, to eat consciously. Ask your body to help you recognize when you become full.

Put down your utensil between bites.

It takes about twenty minutes for the brain and belly to determine *satiety,* or fullness. Putting down your spoon, fork, or chopsticks causes you to slow down and chew, which activates the digestion process and helps your body to pay attention.

Practice *hara hachi bu.*

In the ancient Indian tradition of Ayurveda, the stomach is regarded as a cooking pot, and the digestive metabolism—*agni,* in Sanskrit—fires up that pot. When a cook makes a pot of soup, they have to leave space at the top of the pot, or else the *agni* doesn't properly circulate, and the soup cooks unevenly. The same is true in our digestion. If we overeat, we can't digest properly, and that produces what in Ayurveda is called *ama,* toxic by-products that give birth to degenerative disease. The practice of mindful eating means reconnecting to that moment when our belly and brain say, in unison, "Enough."

The Japanese rule of mindful eating is *hara hachi bu,* or "Eight parts out of ten full." While putting down your utensil, see if you can find that place where you are just full but not stuffed. Don't worry if you can't tell right away; keep practicing and reaffirming your desire to know, and it will come.

Take food with self-confidence.

Allow yourself to enjoy your food wholeheartedly. So often we eat from a place of conflicting emotions: "I want it. I know I shouldn't have it. Who cares? I want it anyway!" What would it be like for you if, instead of saying to yourself, "I'll never eat cake," you could come to a place of having a purely free choice about eating the cake, and either enjoy it wholeheartedly or else let it be?

Take food in one place.

In the Zen tradition there's a saying, "When you eat, just eat; when you sit, just sit." The ideal posture of eating is sitting comfortably, with your focus on the food. If, by contrast, we're eating while driving, in the Ayurvedic view that combination increases *vata,* or wind, which can blow out the *agni* of your digestive fire.

When we take food in one place, we might first encounter boredom, discomfort, and the strong impulse to check our email or read the paper. If this is so for you, I invite you to lean in to the sharp edge of those feelings. You probably won't die from eating without diversion. Any process of healing demands of us that we enter the sanctuary of such feelings without needing to push them away. Breathing through the boredom and discomfort, we discover not only that we can survive but also that we meet a part of ourselves that has been waiting for us for a long, long time.

Enjoy your food.

Here you are, at the supreme meal of your life. Savor every bite. This moment is your feast.

Let's Do Some Tapping

For lots of us it's easier said than done to eat just until satisfied. If you're someone who struggles with tuning in to your body's satiety cues and would like to shake off the habit of overeating, the following Tapping guide is for you.

Tapping Guide 13.1: "I Eat to Overfull"

SETUP STATEMENT: *Even though I have this habit of eating till I'm over-full, I deeply love and accept myself.* (Say aloud one to three times.)

Top of the head: *This habit of overeating—*

Eyebrow: *I eat way past full.*

Side of the eye: *I just keep eating even though I'm full.*

Under the eye: *I feel like such a pig.*

Under the nose: *I can't stop.*

Under the mouth: *All this overeating—*

Collarbone: *I feel so ashamed by it.*

Under arm: *I wish I could figure out how to stop.*

Top of the head: *This overeating—*

Eyebrow: *Some part of me is in a panic.*

Side of the eye: *Maybe I'm afraid there isn't enough,*

Under the eye: *Or there never will be enough.*

Under the nose: *This panicky part of me that overeats,*

Under the mouth: *And everything connected to that part of me—*

Collarbone: *I wonder what's driving this.*

Under arm: *This panic and fear I feel with my food.*

Top of the head: *Can I love myself even with this?*

Eyebrow: *Can I slow down the panic for even a moment?*

Side of the eye: *And be kind to myself?*

Under the eye: *Give myself some understanding?*

Under the nose: *What if I could slow down the panic?*

Under the mouth: *Tune in to my body?*

Collarbone: *Let my body tell me?*

Under arm: *Maybe it can be safe to stop when I'm full.*

Top of the head: *I don't know if it's possible,*

Eyebrow: *But I'm open to it.*

Side of the eye: *And as I open to this possibility,*

Under the eye: *I allow the panic to slow down.*

Under the nose: *It's safe to just eat what I need,*

Under the mouth: *To make friends with my body,*

Collarbone: *To love and appreciate myself—*

Under arm: *Exactly where I'm at.*

Take a nice deep breath. Check in with your initial distress level—is it higher, lower, or about the same? Keep repeating rounds of Tapping until you feel relief.

Do you have a secret addiction to junk food that you feel ashamed of? You know how bad it is for you and the planet, but you just can't stop? Fear not—help is on the way in the following Tapping guide.

Tapping Guide 13.2: "I'm Addicted to Junk Food"

SETUP STATEMENT: *Even though I have this secret junk-food addiction, and I feel really ashamed about it, I deeply love and completely accept myself.* (Say aloud one to three times.)

Top of the head: *This junk-food addiction—*

Eyebrow: *I feel so ashamed.*

Side of the eye: *I can't bear the thought of anyone seeing me eat this food.*

Under the eye: *I know I shouldn't eat it,*

Under the nose: *But I can't help it.*

Under the mouth: *I'm so addicted and so ashamed.*

Collarbone: *It's really horrible.*

Under arm: *I'd die if anyone found out about this.*

Top of the head: *This junk-food addiction,*

Eyebrow: *And everything it means to me—*

Side of the eye: *All this intense shame I feel about it—*

Under the eye: *It makes me want to die of shame.*

Under the nose: *It feels like the worst thing in the world.*

Under the mouth: *But is it?*

Collarbone: *Am I really such a horrible person*

Under arm: *Because I have this addiction?*

Top of the head: *Can I find any part of me*

Eyebrow: *That can send love to this addiction?*

Side of the eye: *I'm in so much pain.*

Under the eye: *Can I send love to the pain?*

Under the nose: *My secret junk-food addiction*

Under the mouth: *And everything I think it means about me—*

Collarbone: *Can I love myself even with this?*

Under arm: *Am I willing to allow this addiction to heal?*

Top of the head: *I don't have to know how that could happen.*

Eyebrow: *I just know that I want to heal.*

Under the eye: *I want to invite a bigger spiritual energy*

Under the nose: *To help me heal this.*

Under the mouth: *The God of My Understanding—*

Collarbone: *Whatever and wherever you are—*

Under arm: *I invite you to help me heal this right now.*

Take a nice deep breath. Check in with your initial distress level—is it higher, lower, or about the same? Keep repeating rounds of Tapping until you feel relief.

Abraham Lincoln once asked, "Do I not destroy my enemies when I make them my friends?" In the next chapter, let me help you discover the hidden gifts that your struggles with food have given you while raising your vibration to fulfill your heart's truest desires.

To tap along with audio recordings of this and other Tapping guides, visit www.marcellafriel.com/taptasteheal.

14

Making Friends with Success

Never forget that you are one of a kind. Never forget that if there weren't any need for you in all your uniqueness to be on this earth, you wouldn't be here in the first place. And never forget, no matter how overwhelming life's challenges and problems seem to be, that one person can make a difference in the world. In fact, it is always because of one person that all the changes that matter in the world come about. So be that one person.

—R. BUCKMINSTER FULLER

IN FEBRUARY 2014, as I was picking through the wreckage that my life had become in Sonoma, California, and wondering how to rebuild, I received clear "guidance" in the wee morning hours following a night of brutal insomnia. The guidance was prompting me to spend that summer in a tiny mountain town in the Sangre de Cristo Mountains of Southern Colorado. I had been to this little town several times before and felt called by the powerful land, the dear old friends who live nearby, and a meditation teacher I had been connecting to via podcast over the winter. I had no money. My business was just getting started. And I was going … *where* for the summer?

If there's one thing I've learned in my fifty-seven years on this earth, however, it's to heed the call of the heart, unreasonable though it might be. When I deny that call because I can't predict how things will work out, I gnaw on regret and wonder, "What would have happened if I had …?" So in mid-June of that year I headed east on Highway 50, "the loneliest road in America," with fear and doubt riding shotgun as my traveling companions. I might as well have been driving off a flat earth.

After a two-week silent meditation retreat and another few weeks visiting friends, I received a call from a client who wanted to work with me. Then another. It was like the drip-drip-drip of rain that presages a deluge. Those first few clients were the early bloomers in a garden that has since proliferated a riot of happy flowers.

Five years later, I'm living in that small town, helping women around the world love and forgive themselves, their food, and their figure while being blessed with more abundance—financial and otherwise—than I ever imagined possible. I am standing at the gateway of a life that is truly beyond my wildest dreams. If I had shrugged off that initial guidance, I might still be wringing my hands in California, wondering how I was going to pay next month's electricity bill.

What callings from your heart have you been afraid to face? Have you been using food to suppress or deny the deeper part of you that knows? A bigger life awaits you just on the other side of your fear. Take my hand. Let's walk through this together.

Want What You Want

In my work with clients and students, I've found it consistently curious that the women who can't curb their urges for Dairy Queen also have no idea of what they really want. Or let me put it another way: they *know* what they want, but they don't let themselves *want* what they want.

This used to puzzle me. Until I got it—when we don't give ourselves what we truly desire, we resort to lower-level compensatory desires that don't satisfy us. Desire is an essential part of life. Flowers desire to grow. Rivers desire to flow to the ocean. Mothers desire to nurse their young. But in a world that's become addicted to self-indulgence, we're told that true desire is selfish. If we're focused on fulfilling our own dreams before taking care of others, we must be self-centered. Certain religious traditions have convinced us that desire is inherently sinful.

No wonder we reach for the cookies and chips. Because the truth is, when we don't abide by the truth of our heart and fulfill our true desires, that energy goes underground and resurfaces as self-soothing/self-harming behaviors.

What have you been longing for but not allowed yourself to have? What have you wanted to want but dared not dream about? If you've been struggling with food and body-love issues, I'm gonna guess that you've put those desires on hold until you're "better": "I'll start dating again when I'm the right body size." "I'll open my artist studio after I lose this weight." "I can't bear to go to belly-dance class right now because I'm too heavy." Or, as my client Madeleine expressed in a group teleconference call, "My weight is holding me back creatively. I want to start a business, so the weight has been one of these conditions that I've placed on my own success—you know, 'I'll be successful when I'm thin' and all that. Last week when I went to get some photos taken, I was so distraught because it was going to capture me at my highest weight ever."

Holding your dreams hostage while striving to be "perfect" or "better" only ensures that everything stays right where it is. I want to suggest to you that it's the other way around. Put your dreams first, and your naturally perfect body size will follow. I invite you, challenge you, and encourage you to place one or both hands on your heart and ask yourself: if you've fallen prey to "Someday I'm gonna …" or "I'd like to, but …" what part of *now* is not the right time to get started?

Stepping In to Your Ordination

Why am I pressing you on this? Because you, as a child of Mother Nature, must express your creativity. According to medical intuitive Caroline Myss, "Creativity is by far one of the most misunderstood currents of life that runs through the human experience…. Creativity is a word we give to the life force. Creativity is an essential essence of life. You are born to create. You can't stop it. The experience of human life is the experience of thought flowing into form, of spirit flowing into matter. When you have a blockage in creativity … it does manifest in illnesses, one of which is the inability to lose weight…. You are holding on to energies that are wanting to be born."[1]

Creativity flows best when we are living our lives from what Dr. Myss calls our *ordination,* our higher purpose. Ordination is the Universe's response to your very authentic question, "What am I here on this earth to do?"

Our ordination is not necessarily what we do for money. The range of possibilities is as vast as the ordinations themselves. Perhaps your ordination is to create beautiful environments where people walk in and immediately feel relaxed. Perhaps you are ordained to bring optimism to everyone you know. Or your ordination is to run a loving home and raise amazing children. Or you could have an ordination like Katherine Coleman Goble Johnson's, a NASA employee (and an African American woman in the 1950s Deep South) whose mathematical trajectory calculations enabled John Glenn to be the first US astronaut to orbit the earth.[2]

It could be anything. What matters is that it's authentic to you. Your ordination is your divine calling, the thing you must do for your life to be meaningful. It might also be the thing that most scares you.

Recognizing Goal Traumas

When clients and students come to work with me, I ask them, "Have you ever been at your ideal weight? What was going on in your life at the time?" I routinely receive answers such as these:

- "I went through a big fitness and weight loss kick after my second child was born, lost a ton of weight, and stayed at my ideal for about eight months, then started gaining again when major stress hit."

- "I slimmed down a lot just in time for my wedding, then immediately afterward found out that my husband had been cheating with one of my bridesmaids. After that, I ballooned up to the highest I'd ever been."

- "I hit my ideal weight and sustained it during the year I trained to run my first marathon. Then two weeks before the event, I twisted my ankle. I was completely devastated, never took up running again, and gained all my weight back."

When you work hard toward realizing a big dream only to have it fail, and you feel extremely reticent about ever trying again, chances are you're carrying a goal trauma.[3] Goal trauma occurs when, despite all your efforts, things don't work out. You not only suffer the loss of that dream; you might also take major hits in other areas of your life: financial loss, dissolution of your marriage, loss of your reputation, and so on.

In response to such devastation, you mean-talk yourself when you think about that experience, saying things like, "What an idiot I was!" or "How could I have been so stupid?" or "What was I thinking?"

Goal traumas can make you approach new desires with deep trepidation. You procrastinate, you quit halfway, or you sabotage your progress, as I discussed in chapter 4. When you carry goal trauma, you trust yourself less, you trust other people less, and you trust the universe less. You doubt that things could ever go your way. You think, "Everyone else might capable of succeeding, but people like me can't break through like that."

Sometimes goal traumas come through the generational line. We carry unconscious guilt over the failures of our parents, grandparents, and ancestors that limits how successful we feel we're allowed to be. In my own case, it took years of Tapping work and spiritual practice to establish deep in my cell tissue that I am not the failures of my parents or the limitations of my tribe. As that truth settled into my being, I was able not only to enjoy success on my own terms but also to energetically send the merit of that success back upstream to them and trust that, wherever they are in their journey, they will receive collateral benefit from my happiness.

Clearing Goal Traumas

Tapping is an excellent tool to heal the emotional ravages of goal traumas, as Amelia's story illustrates. Amelia's daughter, who had been a straight-up A-plus kid her whole life, was now, in her early twenties, lapsing into the same acting-out behaviors that Amelia's ex (and her daughter's father) had demonstrated: drinking, drugs, lying, stealing, and so on. The heartache Amelia felt watching her daughter's downward spiral brought up all of the regret she thought she had resolved around marrying her husband in the first place. She exclaimed through choking tears, "I saved myself for him! I thought it would be wonderful, like it is in the movies. He was so not worth it! And now here's my daughter, taking after him!"

How can we use Tapping to heal monumental regrets such as these?

- *Honor the grief.* Sometimes the grief is so intense there are no words to say. Amelia and I spent a good twenty minutes Tapping together while she cried the tears that had been dammed up for decades.

🐚 *Allow someone to witness you.* Amelia had tried Tapping on her own around this issue, but it wasn't until she felt the presence of a compassionate observer sharing the pain that she was able to touch and release it at a deeper level.

🐚 *Let it rip.* I encouraged Amelia, while Tapping, to scream, shout, cuss, and vocalize everything that her body was holding. While Tapping, she shouted, "How could I have been so dumb?" "What an idiot I was!" And then this: "I wanted it to be like the movies. And instead I married f*cking Joe! How could I have married such an asshole jerk?" As she tapped on and verbalized these last two sentences, Amelia's sobs suddenly turned into peals of laughter. We tapped and laughed and tapped and laughed, saying, "Oops!" "Well, I guess I blew that one!" "Big f*cking oops, huh?" We laughed until our stomachs hurt. After that round of Tapping, Amelia's distress plummeted from a 10 to a 0.

🐚 *Acknowledge your strength.* Once the painful emotions associated with the trauma have been released, it's good to inventory your resilience. However traumatic the loss might have been, however heavy the grief, the truth is that you did survive. How do I know that? Because if the pain had totally taken you out, you wouldn't be reading these words right now.

In Amelia's case, she was able to give herself credit for all the ways she showed up to make the marriage work and marshaled her strength to set loving, appropriate boundaries with her daughter. Two days after our Tapping session, Amelia sent me this message:

> Just wanted to drop a line and let you know I feel soooooo good today!! Wow that belly laugh was amazing. I feel *freeeeee!* That was a ton of bricks to unload. I feel lighter, clearer, and have a spring in my step.

> I talked with my daughter today and apologized for how I handled my immediate reaction to her. And her dad and I had a good talk tonight about how we would communicate on checking in with her progress going forward. *Wild!*

When we face and heal our traumas, we see that, no matter how devastating, each trauma contains the potential for some gift, some blessing, and some lesson. We learn something we wouldn't have otherwise learned; fortunate circumstances emerge from the rubble; we discover a deeper level of belonging to the human family. If you've ever looked back on a past misfortune and thought, "Wow, if that terrible thing hadn't happened, then this great new thing wouldn't have happened," then you know what I mean.

Just as Mother Nature often positions a poisonous plant to grow right alongside its antidote, so it is that our worst traumas often contain within them the very medicine we need to heal.

We Need Your Light

When we live the lives we are meant to live—when we feel fulfilled, purposeful, and of service to our world—we usually feel happy and satisfied, whatever our circumstances. This is why stepping in to our ordination is essential. On a personal level, connecting to our authentic, purposeful place on this planet and manifesting the activity that comes from it release the same feel-good chemicals in your brain that you used to get from binge eating.[4] This is an important piece of healing your relationship with food. It actually changes your brain to follow your path of success.

On a social level, we—Mother Earth and all her children—need your light to shine. It's no secret that our global society and our planet are in crisis. If you examine that crisis more deeply, you will see millions of people denying the truth of who they are, doing what they think they should be doing rather than what their hearts and souls are calling them to do. The more we collectively suppress our ordination, the more we contribute to the demise of society and the degradation of our planet.

Your unique vision contains powerful medicine for our world that only you can administer. Your job—if I may be so bold as to say this—is not to question it or to wonder, "How could I ever do *that?*" Your job is to become an aligned and congruent vessel through which your true purpose flows.

Be—Do—Have

I remember vividly the moment I had achieved the success I desired in my business. It was during a conversation in which Dawn Copeland, my business mentor, invited me into a deeper and significantly more expensive level of work with her. Every cell in my body knew it was the right move for me. I had no idea how I was going to pay for it. I felt like Indiana Jones at the edge of the cliff, staring into the abyss and having no choice but to take a leap of faith.[5]

I said yes.

Just as the crystal bridge appeared the moment Indiana stepped out into that abyss, I knew, in the moment I said yes to my mentor, that I had said yes to my success. And like that crystal bridge, all the resources I needed to walk step by step toward that success appeared—and continue to appear—in their own perfect and miraculous time.

Genuine success doesn't occur the day you make a million bucks or hit the ideal number on the scale. Success begins with finding your inner congruence—in other words, *being* the success—long before the outer manifestation occurs. You know you're congruent with your vision of success when you feel comfortable picturing yourself having it. You feel certain in your bones that it's just a matter of time until it shows up, and there's no rush, no panic, and no what ifs.

My client Madeleine, whom I mentioned earlier, didn't let her apprehension about her body weight diminish her drive to build her business. She chose instead to be the success she was seeking: "I want to remove it as an excuse. I'm really eager to get balanced, I love great food, and I'm excited that I now have a framework for moving forward in health. My business will be a very intuitive business, so I feel that my body is a tuning instrument. The more open I am, the more success and creative expression I'll have."

A good way to jump-start the process of being the success is to start playing the part: "How would a successful person dress for this event?" "How would a successful person walk down this street?" "How would a successful person order their green juice at the juice bar?" and so on. Try the success on for size and see how it fits. As you cultivate your congruence with *being,* you naturally begin *doing* the things that will bring that success closer to you.

Finally, allow yourself to *have.* When you allow yourself to become congruent with what you desire, when you take action to move your energy in that direction, and when you release stuck emotions and limiting beliefs as you go, there inevitably comes the day when the gates open for you, and you *arrive.* When your success comes in this way—by being, doing, and having—you recognize it as a dear old friend who's been at your side all along.

Keep It by Giving It Away

Finally, the best way to keep your success is to give it away. By this, I don't mean codependently taking care of everyone else until your cup runs dry. What I mean is that our ordination is not for us alone. When we remember that we are here on Mother Earth both to fulfill ourselves and to serve others, we're inoculated against self-centered fear and self-pity—two deadly energies that can cause us to reach for our trigger foods.

When we genuinely serve and help others, our focus shifts away from obsessing about our shortcomings and toward the joy of giving with no expectation of return. We raise our self-esteem by finding that we have something valuable to offer that someone else needs. We dust off inner resources that have been moldering away inside our self-preoccupation. We feel good because we make someone else's day—or year—or life.

Giving it away can take the form of direct action. It can also take the form of prayer, of filling up your cup from that inexhaustible source I mentioned in the previous chapter and sharing the overflow by energetically wishing, "May all beings be happy; may all beings be healed," starting with those closest to you whom you love most dearly, then expanding out to those whom you feel neutral about, then to those toward whom you feel aversion or animosity, and, finally, to all beings everywhere, on planet earth and far, far beyond.

The more you give in this manner, the more blessings, miracles, and synchronicities shower back upon you. In the words of American futurist R. Buckminster Fuller, "You can rest assured that if you devote your time and attention to the highest advantage of others, the Universe will support you, always and only in the nick of time."[6]

Are You Willing?

Well, dear reader, we've come to the end of our journey, or at least this leg of it. I want to invite you to find a quiet space within yourself. If you like, you can place your hands on your heart and take three deep, conscious breaths. When your mind has shifted into that quieter space, ask yourself, from your heart: "Is hating my body still an option for me? Or am I ready to put that to rest? Am I willing to die to my old identity as someone who can't, who doesn't deserve, who is defined by failure and shame? Am I willing, in this very moment, to say yes to unconditional self-love, to say yes to forgiveness, to say yes to valuing and cherishing myself exactly as I am?"

Well done, brave one. I welcome you with open arms as you cross the threshold into your wild new adventure.

In closing, I leave you with this blessing from the late master mythologist Joseph Campbell: "We have not even to risk the adventure alone, for the heroes of all time have gone before us. The labyrinth is thoroughly known; we have only to follow the thread of the hero's path. And where we had thought to find an abomination, we shall find a god. And where we had thought to slay another, we shall slay ourselves. And where we had thought to travel outward, we shall come to the center of our own existence. And where we had thought to be alone, we shall be with all the world."[7]

Let's Do Some Tapping

If you know you have unresolved goal trauma, use the following questions to help you figure out what you need to tap on:

- What happened that wasn't supposed to happen? What should have happened instead?

- What judgments do I have about myself and others about it?

- How is it hindering me around moving forward?

Then tap along with this Tapping guide:

Tapping Guide 14.1: Healing Goal Trauma

SETUP STATEMENT: *Even though I still feel traumatized over what happened, and I feel like a total failure, I choose to love myself right where I'm at.* (Say aloud one to three times.)

Top of the head: *I still feel horrible about it.*

Eyebrow: *What a disaster!*

Side of the eye: *I feel like such a failure.*

Under the eye: *All that hard work for nothing.*

Under the nose: *Such a colossal failure.*

Under the mouth: *How could I have been so dumb?*

Collarbone: *It's still overwhelming just to think about it.*

Under arm: *I can hardly stand it.*

Top of the head: *It shouldn't have turned out that way.*

Eyebrow: *I worked so hard.*

Side of the eye: *All for nothing.*

Under the eye: *I can't stop beating myself up about it.*

Under the nose: *I'll never forgive myself.*

Under the mouth: *It's so incredibly painful to remember it.*

Collarbone: *All this disappointment.*

Under arm: *It's totally overwhelming.*

Top of the head: *How can I ever move forward again?*

Eyebrow: *Part of me wants to curl up and die.*

Side of the eye: *But the truth is—*

Under the eye: *I did the best I could at the time.*

Under the nose: *And I want to honor that.*

Under the mouth: *Cut myself a little slack.*

Collarbone: *It sucks that it was such a failure,*

Under arm: *But at least I stepped up to the plate.*

Top of the head: *I learned a lot from this experience.*

Eyebrow: *It was a painful lesson, for sure.*

Side of the eye: *But I didn't totally crumble.*

Under the eye: *I'm wiser for the experience.*

> **Under the nose:** *I totally honor everything that happened.*
>
> **Under the mouth:** *And it's okay to let it go,*
>
> **Collarbone:** *Love and forgive myself,*
>
> **Under arm:** *Take a fresh start and move forward.*

Take a nice deep breath. Check in with your initial distress level—is it higher, lower, or about the same? Keep repeating rounds of Tapping until you feel relief.

If you know, theoretically, that you're supposed to love your body as it is, but there's a deeper part of you that really is waiting for the weight to disappear before you pursue your dreams, this Tapping guide is for you.

Tapping Guide 14.2: "Life Begins after I Lose the Weight"

SETUP STATEMENT: Even though I feel like life begins after I lose the weight, I deeply love and accept myself. (Say aloud one to three times.)

Top of the head: *Life begins after I lose the weight.*

Eyebrow: *I know I'm supposed to love myself where I am—*

Side of the eye: *And all of that stuff.*

Under the eye: *But the truth is—*

Under the nose: *I want to lose this damn weight!*

Under the mouth: *And I'm not moving forward until I do.*

Collarbone: *I can't move forward until this weight is gone.*

Under arm: *And that's just how it is.*

Top of the head: *I can't have what I want*

Eyebrow: *Until the weight is gone.*

Side of the eye: *When I'm thin, I'll deserve.*

Under the eye: *When I'm thin, I'll be happy and successful.*

Under the nose: *There's no other way.*

Under the mouth: *Someday I'm gonna lose this weight.*

Collarbone: *And then my life will fall into place.*

Under arm: *And all my problems will be gone.*

Top of the head: *Is that really true?*

Eyebrow: *Is it absolutely true?*

Side of the eye: *I wonder how this thought serves me—*

Under the eye: *That my life begins after I lose the weight.*

Under the nose: *Is it really true?*

Under the mouth: *Maybe some part of me likes things as they are.*

Collarbone: *Maybe the weight gives me an excuse*

Under arm: *To stay invisible and not show up.*

Top of the head: *Maybe I'm scared to move forward.*

Eyebrow: *Whatever it is—*

Side of the eye: *I want to be my own best friend right now.*

Under the eye: *I want to be kind to myself.*

Under the nose: *And I want to be honest with myself.*

Under the mouth: *As best I can in this moment,*

Collarbone: *I want to clear whatever's really in the way*

Under arm: *Of me living the life I desire.*

Take a nice deep breath. Check in with your initial distress level—is it higher, lower, or about the same? Keep repeating rounds of Tapping until you feel relief.

Tapping Guide 14.3: Master Manifester Tapping Guide

This is a fun Tapping guide for manifesting what you truly desire. This guide will help you raise your vibration and get you into the feeling space of being the success you want to manifest in your life.

Let's begin as I like to begin, by placing your hands on your heart and taking three deep, conscious breaths. While your hands are on your heart center, continue breathing normally and allow your energy to settle into a deeper level of awareness. Take as much time as you need to get into this space.

As you sit in the stillness, bring to mind something creative you have been wanting for a long time. Perhaps you want to begin painting again, or maybe you want to start a new business, or maybe you want to plant a garden—whatever it is, allow yourself to connect at the heart level with what it is you really want for yourself.

Once you have it, say your desire aloud to yourself: "I want to plant a vegetable garden this next spring." As you follow the Tapping guide below, insert your desire in the places where I indicate in the phrases that follow—I used "achieve my desire" as a placeholder for where you should use your own words to state what you desire.

Begin by tapping on the side of your hand and say aloud three times: "*Even though I haven't always achieved my desire* [use your own words here], *I deeply love and completely accept myself.*"

Top of the head: *I haven't always achieved my desire.*

Eyebrow: *I want to always achieve my desire.*

Side of the eye: *I choose to always achieve my desire.*

Under the eye: *I love to always achieve my desire, because ...* [Continuing to tap under the eye, say aloud to yourself all the reasons why you love to always achieve this desire.]

Under the nose: *If I were always to achieve my desire, my life would look like ...* [Again, continuing to tap under the nose, either verbalize or just bring to mind all the positive images you associate with achieving this particular desire.]

Under the mouth: *When I achieve my desire, I will hear other people say ...* [Continuing to tap under the mouth, what would you expect to hear other people say about you? Say those things aloud.] And I would hear myself say ... [What would you be saying to yourself about yourself?]

Collarbone: *In order to achieve my desire, the actions I need to take are ...* [Continuing to tap on the collarbone, verbalize the actions you need to take with as much detail as possible. What are the actions you need to take to achieve your desire?]

Under the arm: *If I were to always achieve my desire, I would feel ...* [Continuing to tap under the arm, get into the feeling space of how it will feel to achieve this. Say those words aloud and allow the feelings to move through your entire body.]

Now here are some new tapping points to use that we haven't used yet. You're going to tap on each finger on one hand (it doesn't matter which one) with the fingers of the other hand. You're going to tap on the side of the finger closest to your torso, on the lower corner where the nail joins the flesh.

Thumb: Choose an image that you associate with achieving your desire. Make sure you yourself are in that image. Once you have a clear image, allow it to hover in front of you; then allow it to float up and hover over the top of your head. When you're ready, imagine that you can open the top of your head and allow this image to pour down into your brain.

Index finger: Allow this image to swirl through your brain and imagine all the neural pathways in your brain reconfiguring to make this image your new reality. Let it literally wash your brain and repattern it so that this really becomes your new reality.

Middle finger: Allow this image to melt and stream and pour down through your entire body, from the top of your head, through your neck and shoulders, and down your arms, your torso, and your legs and feet. Connect to the sense of success, achievement, and joy embedded in this energy. Send a signal to every cell in your body that this success is your new reality.

Ring finger: Take this image into your heart. Let this image really abide there.

Baby finger: Make the colors around the image really vivid and clear. See the image with as much clarity as you can create. Get in touch with all the positive emotions you associate with this image and also connect to any sense perceptions. What are you hearing, seeing, feeling, smelling, tasting?

Wrist point: Tapping inside your pulse, take a nice strong breath. On the exhale, imagine this image bursting out of your body like rays bursting out of the sun, extending all the way above, below, behind, and in front of you—360 degrees—to the farthest reaches of the universe. Give yourself time to really feel this, so there's a strong sense of this image being out there.

Side of the hand: Bring to mind and say aloud all the people, things, and circumstances you are grateful for in relation to achieving your desire.

Now here's the fun part: do a happy dance! The dance is to seal the new behavior with positive emotions.

Remember that what we focus on expands. Do this every day for twenty-eight days, and you will repattern your brain to welcome in and achieve what you desire.

Tapping Guide 14.4: Meeting Your Future Self

This is a Tapping guide to help you become congruent with the *you* of your future, who has already healed their relationship with their food, who has mastered self-care, and who is now living their life at a body weight that feels completely comfortable to them.

Visualizing the results you want as if they are already occurring sets up your brain patterns to make that experience your new reality. Professional athletes, public speakers, and other performers have known this for a long time. They rehearse the results they want to achieve in their minds first, which enables them to manifest it later.

Begin by tapping on your collarbone point or on any point that feels comfortable to you. Close your eyes and take a few deep, conscious breaths. Allow your body to relax. Bring your attention and your focus inward. If you like, you can focus your energy on your heart center.

From this place of inner focus, imagine yourself in an environment that feels relaxing to you. It could be a room in your house; someplace in nature, like the beach, the woods, or a mountaintop; or a sacred space, like a temple or cave. See yourself there as you are right now. When that feels clear to you, invite your future self into the space with you. This could be yourself one year from now, five years from now, eighteen months from now—whatever time frame you feel it will take you to achieve the results you want to achieve.

It's okay if the image is fuzzy at first. As you breathe and relax, allow the image to become clearer. You might start by noticing the happy, peaceful, and satisfied expression on their face. They are well dressed—radiant—and have let go of all of their stress around food. Their body aligns with their brilliance and light, and they've given themselves permission to shine in the world. This is you in the future, accomplishing what you have set out to accomplish.

(Before we proceed further, check in with yourself to see, on a scale of 1 to 10, with 10 being the highest, how congruent—how possible, realistic, and accessible—this future self feels to you. If your number is less than a 5, I suggest you pause this exercise and tap on yourself with the setup statement, *"Even though I don't feel congruent with the results I'd like to create, I deeply love and accept myself"* and take it from there. Come back to this guide when you feel like you have more congruency with the future self you're creating. If your number is higher than a 5, let's proceed.)

If it feels comfortable to you, allow your future self to take your hand. Tell them, in your words, where you feel like you're struggling to get yourself to where they are now. Imagine that while you're talking to them, they are tapping on the side of your hand while you tap on your own hand. When you're ready, allow your future self in this scenario to tap on you, while you tap on yourself in real time and say aloud the words your future self is saying to you:

SETUP STATEMENT: *Even though you are struggling with* [use your own words], *and you feel* [insert what you are feeling] *about it, I understand, I know where you're at, and I was there too. And I see what a beautiful person you are, and I love you so much, and I am here to help you.* (Say aloud one time.)

Top of the head: *All the struggle you're having,*

Eyebrow: *Everything you're struggling with,*

Side of the eye: *All this struggle,*

Under the eye: *I understand.*

Under the nose: *I see you.*

Under the mouth: *I love you.*

Collarbone: *I am here for you.*

Under arm: *I believe in you.*

Top of the head: *And I know you can do this.*

Eyebrow: *And I am here to help you.*

Side of the eye: *I will do whatever I can for you.*

Under the eye: *I see you.*

Under the nose: *I love you.*

Under the mouth: *I believe in you.*

Collarbone: *I know you can do this.*

Under arm: *I am here to help.*

Take a nice deep breath. Ask your future self to share with you whatever wisdom they have to help you get to where they are. Allow them to counsel you on what you need to let go of—behaviors, emotions, beliefs, habits, and so on. Then ask them what you need to embrace, adopt, and integrate. Again, they could be beliefs, emotions, habits, behaviors. As they are speaking with you, see them beaming, smiling at you, loving you, taking your hands in their hands. Take in their wisdom.

When you're ready, thank them for coming to visit you and allow them to begin to dissolve into a sphere of light of a color that resonates with you. Allow that light to swirl in front of you until it enters into your heart center. As best you can, allow your heart to open, take in that light, and allow it to move through your heart center, softening any places where there might be resistance. Let the light spiral through your chest, all the way up to your shoulders, neck, and head, and all the way down to your pelvic floor, your legs and feet, and let that light keep spiraling around your body until it fills the whole of who you are.

Let every cell in your body know that now you are, in present time, the self of your future that you have been wanting to manifest. You might want to place one or both hands on your heart and allow yourself to be that person. Allow yourself to embody success, well-being, excellent self-care, unconditional self-love. Allow that to be reflected in every part of your body.

When you're ready, see your future self again in your heart center as they appeared to you initially. Take a nice deep breath, and as you exhale, beam that energy out of your body like rays bursting out of the sun, 360 degrees around you, all the way above and all the way below, to the farthest reaches of the Universe. Send it all the way back through your history and all the way through your future, so that the entire quantum field receives and aligns itself with this expression of your highest intention.

Let yourself rest in this space as long as you like. When you're ready, take out your journal and jot down any insights you had from this meditation. Then check in with yourself to see how congruent this future self feels now. Repeat this meditation as needed until that congruence feels solidly established in your being.

To tap along with audio recordings of this and other Tapping guides, visit www.marcellafriel.com/taptasteheal.

Appendix

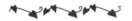

EFT How-to Chart

EFT HOW-TO CHART

Focus on the distress you want to resolve. If you have several issues you want to work on, focus on the one that's most stressful right now.

Assign a Subjective Units of Distress (SUD) to the problem. On a scale of 1 (lowest) to 10 (highest), rate how intense the distress is.

Create a setup statement. "Even though I [state the problem], I deeply love and completely accept myself." Repeat the statement aloud 3 times while tapping on the fleshy part of the outside of the hand with the four fingers of the other hand.

Tap around the points. Tap lightly about five to seven times on each point in the illustration, starting at the top of the head and ending at the underarm point.

While tapping on the points, say aloud to yourself a short reminder phrase to keep the focus on the issue you're tapping on.

Remeasure your SUD level. After you complete a round or two of tapping, re-visit your initial distress. What SUD number would you give it now? If you're not yet at 0, begin the process again. The goal is to get your SUD to 0.

The information in this EFT Chart is not intended to replace qualified medical or psychological advice or treatment. Marcella encourages you to always make your own health decisions with a qualified medical or psychological professional.

paula@paulahansen.com

TAPPING with Marcella

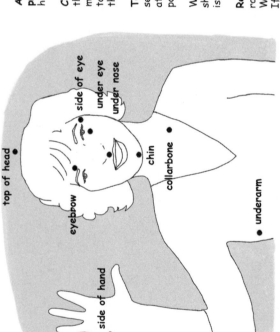

top of head

side of eye
under eye
under nose

eyebrow

chin
collarbone

side of hand

underarm

Marcella Friel
mindful eating mentor for health-conscious women
marcellafriel.com

Notes

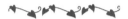

Chapter 1

1 *Merriam-Webster,* s.v. "stress (*n.*)," www.merriam-webster.com/dictionary/stress.

2 Technically, the correct term is *amygdalae,* as there is a pair of tissues rather than one entity. I've chosen here to go with the popular parlance of *amygdala* rather than the technically correct term.

3 Jessica Ortner, *The Tapping Solution: A Woman's Guide to Stressing Less, Weighing Less, and Loving More* (Los Angeles: Hay House, 2014), 5.

4 Matthew Dahlitz, "The Triune Brain," *Neuropsychotherapist,* October 16, 2016, www.neuropsychotherapist.com/the-triune-brain.

5 Peta B. Stapleton, "Selected Works of Peta B. Stapleton," *Bepress,* https://works.bepress.com/peta_stapleton.

6 "30 Years of Thought Field Therapy," *Thought Field Therapy News,* www.rogercallahan.com/news/30-years-of-thought-field-therapy.

7 Ortner, *Tapping Solution,* 8.

Chapter 2

1 Mary Tynes, "Louise Hay on Working through 'Negative Issues,' Childhood Trauma," *Mary Tynes,* www.marytynes.com/2015/09/12/louise-hay-on-working-through-negative-issues-childhood-trauma.

Chapter 3

1 Carl Sandburg, "Fog," www.poetryfoundation.org/poems/45032/fog-56d2245d7b36c.

2 "What Is the Origin of the Word 'Diet'?" *Culinary Lore,* August 26, 2014, www.culinarylore.com/food-history:origin-of-the-word-diet.

3 The Militant Baker: Lose the Bullshit, Liberate Your Body, www.themilitant-baker.com.

4 Quoted in the documentary film *Embrace,* written and directed by Taryn Brumfitt (Glenside, Australia: Southern Light Alliance and the Body Image Movement, 2016), DVD.

5 Alexandra Sifferlin, "The Weight Loss Trap: Why Your Diet Isn't Working," *TIME,* June 5, 2017, http://time.com/magazine/us/4793878/june-5th-2017-vol-189-no-21-u-s.

6 Linda Bacon, Ph.D., https://lindabacon.org.

7 Sandra Aamodt, "Why You Can't Lose Weight on a Diet," *New York Times,* May 6, 2016, www.nytimes.com/2016/05/08/opinion/sunday/why-you-cant-lose-weight-on -a-diet.html.

8 Quoted in the documentary film *Embrace,* written and directed by Taryn Brumfitt.

9 Meredith Melnick, "Global Spread: More People Think 'Fat People Are Lazy,' " *TIME,* March 31, 2011, http://healthland.time.com/2011/03/31/global-spread-more-people -think-fat-people-are-lazy.

10 M. Morris, "10 Frightening Ways We Discriminate Against Fat People," *Listverse,* September 27, 2013, https://listverse.com/2013/09/27/10-frightening-ways-we -discriminate-against-fat-people.

11 Linda Bacon, "Busting Myths on Health and Weight," video, 7:24, https://lindabacon .org/videos/busting-myths-health-weight.

12 Sifferlin, "The Weight Loss Trap."

Chapter 4

1 I want to thank Katherine Woodward Thomas for introducing the concept of a false love identity in her landmark book, *Calling in "the One": Seven Weeks to Attract the Love of Your Life* (New York: Three Rivers Press, 2004). In this section, I borrow from much of her work to flesh out the false food ego.

2 I first learned about vows of loyalty and rebellion from Margaret Lynch in her book *Tapping into Wealth: How Emotional Freedom Techniques (EFT) Can Help You Clear the Path to Making More Money* (New York: Tarcher/Penguin, 2013).

Chapter 5

1 *Merriam-Webster,* s.v. "addiction (*n.*)," www.merriam-webster.com/dictionary /addiction.

2 *Merriam-Webster,* s.v. "compulsion (*n.*)," www.merriam-webster.com/dictionary /compulsion.

3 "Frequently Asked Questions about Food Allergies," *US Food and Drug Administration,* www.fda.gov/Food/IngredientsPackagingLabeling/FoodAllergens /ucm530854.htm

4 If you suspect you do have a food allergy, you might consider keeping a food journal. Write down what you eat and then how you feel twenty minutes later. I did this years ago, when I was living in New York City and eating a lot of bagels. I had no idea that white flour could trigger my anger like nobody's business. I would go to Columbia Bagels at 110th and Broadway and order a whitefish on everything then get on the subway, and I wanted to murder everyone on the train. That awareness helped me to decide not to eat bagels anymore.

5 Julia Child, *My Life in France* (New York: Anchor Books, 2006), 282.

6 United States Department of Agriculture Economic Research Service, FAQs, www.ers.usda.gov/faqs/#Q2.

7 David Zivot, "Is Wheat Genetically Modified?" *Grainstorm Heritage Baking*, June 4, 2017, https://grainstorm.com/blogs/blog/is-wheat-genetically-modified.

8 "A Guide to Grains," *Healthy Beginnings,* September 1, 2012, www.hbmag.com/a-guide-to-grains.

9 Donna Gates, "The Pasteurized Foods You Should Consider Avoiding and the Healthy Reasons Why," *Body Ecology,* https://bodyecology.com/articles/avoid_pasteurized_foods.php.

10 "Homogenization: A Closer Look," www.raw-milk-facts.com/homogenization_T3.html.

11 Emily Benfit, "Think Fat-Free Milk Is Healthy? 6 Secrets You Don't Know About Skim," *Butter Believer,* http://butterbeliever.com/fat-free-dairy-skim-milk-secrets.

12 Kris Gunnars, "How Food Addiction Works," *Healthline,* May 15, 2018, www.healthline.com/nutrition/how-food-addiction-works.

13 *Alcoholics Anonymous: The Story of How Many Thousands of Men and Women Have Recovered from Alcoholism,* 3rd ed. (New York: Alcoholics Anonymous World Services, 1976), 35–37.

14 Nina Martrys, "'Paradise Lost': How the Apple Became the Forbidden Fruit," *NPR,* April 30, 2017, www.npr.org/sections/thesalt/2017/04/30/526069512/paradise-lost-how-the-apple-became-the-forbidden-fruit.

15 Gabor Maté, "The Warm Embrace of Addiction," *Omega,* October 21, 2013, www.eomega.org/article/the-warm-embrace-of-addiction.

Chapter 6

1 Michael Pollan, *Food Rules: An Eater's Manual* (New York: Penguin, 2009), 85.

2 Online Etymology Dictionary, s.v. "Decide (v.)," www.etymonline.com/word/decide.

3 Magalie Lenoir, "Intense Sweetness Surpasses Cocaine Reward," *PLOS One,* August 1, 2017, http://journals.plos.org/plosone/article?id=10.1371/journal.pone.0000698.

Chapter 7

1 Rose Eveleth, "There Are 37.2 Trillion Cells in Your Body," *Smithsonian,* October 24, 2013, www.smithsonianmag.com/smart-news/there-are-372-trillion-cells-in-your -body-4941473.

2 *The Phrase Finder,* "Abracadabra," www.phrases.org.uk/meanings/abracadabra.html.

3 "The Word and Unstruck Sound," *Mythphile,* March 5, 2011, www.mythphile.com /2011/03/the-word-and-unstruck-sound.

4 I learned this perspective in Katherine Woodward Thomas's book, *Calling in "the One": Seven Weeks to Attract the Love of Your Life* (New York: Three Rivers Press, 2004).

5 Kate Wong, "Why Humans Give Birth to Helpless Babies," *Scientific American,* August 28, 2012, https://blogs.scientificamerican.com/observations/why-humans-give-birth -to-helpless-babies.

6 Bruce Lipton, "Are You Programmed at Birth?" *You Can Heal Your Life Articles,* August 17, 2010, www.healyourlife.com/are-you-programmed-at-birth.

7 Robert Scaer, *8 Keys to Body-Brain Balance* (New York: Norton, 2012), http://books. wwnorton.com/books/8-Keys-to-Brain–Body-Balance.

8 "Understanding Trauma with Dr Robert Scaer," YouTube video, 49:35, interview by Craig Weiner, posted by "Craig Weiner, D.C.," June 9, 2015, www.youtube.com /watch?v=85mUMYw2SW4.

9 Kim D'Eramo, with Jessica Ortner, "How to Use EFT Tapping to Rebalance Your Body and Mind to Overcome Autoimmune Disorders." *The Tapping Solution,* www .thetappingsolution.com/autoimmune/overcoming-autoimmune-disorders.php.

10 Sylvia Hartmann, *The Advanced Patterns of EFT* (Eastbourne, U.K.: DragonRising, January 2003), http://qstc.yolasite.com/resources/The%20Advanced%20Patterns %20Of%20Eft.pdf.

11 Paul Zelizer, "Using Tail Enders to Find Core Issues," *The Gary Craig Official EFT Training Centers,* www.emofree.com/articles-ideas/core-issue/tail-ender-eft-article.html.

12 Karl Dawson, with Sasha Allenby, *Matrix Reimprinting Using EFT: Rewrite Your Past, Transform Your Future* (London: Hay House, 2010).

Chapter 8

1 Edward Espe Brown, *Tomato Blessings and Radish Teachings* (New York: Riverhead, 1997), 268.

2 "Saturated Fats: Why All the Hubbub over Coconuts?" *American Heart Association News,* https://news.heart.org/saturated-fats-why-all-the-hubbub-over-coconuts.

3 "Obesity and Overweight," *Centers for Disease Control and Prevention,* www .cdc.gov/nchs/fastats/obesity-overweight.htm.

4 Marion Nestle, *Food Politics: How the Food Industry Influences Nutrition and Health* (Berkeley: University of California Press, 2002), 315–16.

5 Eric Schlosser, *Fast Food Nation: The Dark Side of the All-American Meal* (Boston: Houghton Mifflin, 2001), http://jhampton.pbworks.com/w/file/fetch/51769044 /Fast%20Food%20Nation.pdf.

6 "The Impact of Food Advertising on Childhood Obesity," *American Psychological Association,* www.apa.org/topics/kids-media/food.aspx.

7 Annemarie Colbin, *Food and Healing: How What You Eat Determines Your Health, Your Well-Being, and the Quality of Your Life* (New York: Ballantine, 1986).

8 "Teikei: Putting the Farmer's Face on Food," *Oxfam Australia,* May 8, 2013, www .oxfam.org.au/2013/05/teikei-putting-the-farmers-face-on-food.

9 Pollan, *Food Rules,* 99.

Chapter 9

1 I owe a deep bow of gratitude to my colleague Mary Sheila Gonnella of Occidental Nutrition, whose *Breakfast Report* supplied most of the source material for this section of the chapter.

2 Mind you, I'm not a doctor, and what I'm suggesting here is not a diagnosis. If you're really curious about your hormone levels, go get them tested by a qualified health-care professional.

3 "Weight Loss and Leptin Resistance," *The Gabriel Method,* www.thegabrielmethod .com/audio-leptin-resistance.

4 It's way beyond the scope of this book to get into this issue, but if you'd like a primer on the food industry's big fat lie, please read Sally Fallon and Mary G. Enig, "The Skinny on Fats," *Weston A. Price Foundation,* January 1, 2000, www.westonaprice.org /health-topics/know-your-fats/the-skinny-on-fats.

5 "Tony Robbins—One Millimeter Off," YouTube video, 1:47, posted by "Eric Isaacson," October 7, 2014, www.youtube.com/watch?v=ciJWcURRan0.

Chapter 10

1 Dinitia Smith, "When Flour Power Invaded the Kitchen," *New York Times,* April 14, 2004, www.nytimes.com/2004/04/14/dining/when-flour-power-invaded-the -kitchen.html.

2 Michael Pollan, "Out of the Kitchen, Onto the Couch," *New York Times,* July 29, 2009, www.nytimes.com/2009/08/02/magazine/02cooking-t.html.

3 "The Average American Spends 24 Hours a Week Online," *The Download*, January 23, 2018, www.technologyreview.com/the-download/610045/the-average-american-spends-24-hours-a-week-online.

4 Ornish Lifestyle Medicine, www.ornish.com/proven-program/love-support.

5 Raj Patel, *Stuffed and Starved: The Hidden Battle for the World Food System* (New York: Melville House, 2012).

6 Chögyam Trungpa, *Shambhala: The Sacred Path of the Warrior* (Boston: Shambhala, 1984), 33.

7 Edward Espe Brown, *Tomato Blessings and Radish Teachings* (New York: Riverhead, 1997), 28.

8 Kamikoto, "The Japanese Art to Eating with Your Eyes," *Kamikoto Blog*, January 24, 2018, http://kamikotoblog.com/the-japanese-art-to-eating-with-your-eyes.

Chapter 11

1 Rob Koke, "God of the Valleys, Part 3: Valleys Others Create," Sermon, Shoreline Christian Church, Austin, TX, no date.

2 *Merriam-Webster*, s.v. "forgive (*v.*)," www.merriam-webster.com/dictionary/forgive.

3 Caroline Myss. *Why People Don't Heal*. Audio Recording. Boulder, CO: Sounds True.

4 *Alcoholics Anonymous: The Story of How Many Thousands of Men and Women Have Recovered from Alcoholism*, 3rd ed. (New York: Alcoholics Anonymous World Services, 1976), 552.

Chapter 12

1 Jerry Mander, *In the Absence of the Sacred: The Failure of Technology and the Survival of the Indian Nations* (San Francisco: Sierra Club Books, 1991), 97.

2 Teen Futures Media Network, University of Washington, http://depts.washington.edu/thmedia/teenfutures/index.html.

3 Brumfitt, *Embrace*.

4 "Eating Disorders: Body Image and Advertising," *Healthy Place*, May 30, 2017, www.healthyplace.com/eating-disorders/articles/eating-disorders-body-image-and-advertising.

5 Paul Hamburg, "The Media and Eating Disorders: Who Is Most Vulnerable?" Public Forum: Culture, Media, and Eating Disorders, Harvard Medical School, 1998, www.healthyplace.com/eating-disorders/articles/eating-disorders-body-image-and-advertising.

6 Brené Brown, "Listening to Shame," TED2012, www.ted.com/talks/brene_brown_listening_to_shame.

7 Byron Katie, "The Work of Byron Katie: An Introduction," *The Work*, http://thework.com/sites/thework/downloads/Little%20Book.pdf.

8 "Brené Brown: Perfectionism Is the 20-Ton Shield We Use to Protect Ourselves (Video)," *Huffpost,* October 5, 2013, www.huffingtonpost.com/2013/10/05/brene-brown-perfectionism-shame-oprah_n_4045358.html.

9 For more on the topic of "always striving but never arriving," see Margaret Lynch, *Tapping into Wealth: How Emotional Freedom Techniques (EFT) Can Help You Clear the Path to Making More Money* (New York: Tarcher/Penguin, 2013).

10 Quoted in the documentary film *Straight/Curve: Redefining Body Image,* written and directed by Jenny McQuaile (New York: Beautiful Curve, Salty Features, 2017), www.straightcurvefilm.com.

11 Wikipedia, s.v. "Aerie (American Eagle Outfitters)," https://en.wikipedia.org/wiki/Aerie_(American_Eagle_Outfitters)#History

12 Quoted in the film *Straight/Curve: Redefining Body Image*, by Jenny McQuaile.

13 "Narcissus," *Greek Mythology,* www.greekmythology.com/Myths/Mortals/Narcissus/narcissus.html.

14 Raskolnick, "Ameinias and Narcissus," *My Pillow Book,* September 9, 2006, https://raskolnick.wordpress.com/2006/09/09/ameinias-and-narcissus.

15 "The person you really need to marry | Tracy McMillan | TEDxOlympicBlvdWomen," YouTube video, 13:58, posted by TEDx Talks, February 7, 2014, www.youtube.com/watch?v=P3fIZuW9P_M.

Chapter 13

1 Trungpa, *Shambhala,* 56.

2 *Food Wastage Footprint: Impacts on Natural Resources*, PDF Document, United Nations Food and Agriculture Organization, 2013, www.fao.org/docrep/018/i3347e/i3347e.pdf.

3 Somini Sengupta, "How Much Food Do We Waste? Probably More Than You Think," *New York Times,* December 12, 2017, www.nytimes.com/2017/12/12/climate/food-waste-emissions.html.

4 Lynne Twist, with Pedram Shojai, bonus interview for the film *Prosperity,* https://well.org/prosperity.

5 This is a super-complex issue having to do with government food policies that subsidize the overproduction of cheap commodity crops, that turn into cheap processed foods available everywhere, that turn into visceral fat and degenerative disease in the bodies of those who consume them, that all adds up to an overwhelming situation for Mother Earth and her children. A great book on this topic, by the way, is Raj Patel's *Stuffed and Starved: The Hidden Battle for the World's Food System* (Brooklyn, NY: Melville House, 2012). Nonetheless, I raise these issues because I feel passionately that it's important to understand the maze of social, political, and global factors that contribute to your personal suffering around food choices and food habits. The industrial food system likes to tell us

that our struggles are just a lack of individual willpower. That is by no means the whole story. It's absolutely our responsibility to take care of our health—but it's not our fault that we're in this predicament.

6 "Bottomless Bowls: Why Visual Portions of Food Size May Influence Intake," Food & Brand Lab, Cornell University, http://foodpsychology.cornell.edu/content /bottomless-bowls-why-visual-cues-portion-size-may-influence-intake.

7 Frances Moore Lappé, *Diet for a Small Planet* (New York: Ballantine, 1971).

8 Mary Duenwald, "A Conversation with Marion Nestle: An 'Eat More' Message for a Fattened America," *New York Times,* February 19, 2002, www.nytimes.com/2002/02/19 /health/a-conversation-with-marion-nestle-an-eat-more-message-for-a-fattened -america.html.

9 Tara Parker-Pope, "Well: Michael Pollan Offers 64 Ways to Eat Food," *New York Times,* January 8, 2010, http://well.blogs.nytimes.com/2010/01/08/michael-pollan -offers-64-ways-to-eat-food.

10 Sengupta, "How Much Food Do We Waste?"

11 Chögyam Trungpa, *Meditation in Action* (Boston: Shambhala, 1969), 23.

12 Bernie Glassman and Rick Fields, *Instructions to the Cook: A Zen Master's Advice on Living a Life That Matters* (New York: Bell Tower, 1996), 10.

Chapter 14

1 Caroline Myss, *The Three Levels of Power and How to Use Them* (Boulder, CO: Sounds True, 1998).

2 Michael Neufeld, "Katherine Johnson, Hidden Figures, and John Glenn's Flight," *Smithsonian National Air and Space Museum,* February 20, 2017, https://airandspace .si.edu/stories/editorial/glenn-johnson-hidden-figures.

3 I learned about goal traumas in Margaret Lynch's wonderful book, *Tapping Into Wealth: How Emotional Freedom Techniques (EFT) Can Help You Clear the Path to Making More Money* (New York: Tarcher/Penguin, 2013).

4 Thai Nguyen, "How to Hack Your Brain Chemicals to Be More Productive," *Entrepreneur,* August 4, 2016, www.entrepreneur.com/video/279853.

5 "Indiana Jones and the Last Crusade," YouTube video, 2:09, the leap of faith scene, posted by "C. Catherine," September 7, 2010, www.youtube.com/watch?v=xFntFdEGgws.

6 AZ Quotes, www.azquotes.com/quote/571592.

7 Joseph Campbell Quotable Quotes, www.goodreads.com/quotes/37475-the-hero -path-we-have-not-even-to-risk-the.

Index

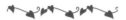

C

D

E

F

About the Author

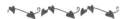

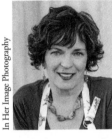

MARCELLA FRIEL is a mindful eating mentor and natural foods chef who helps health-conscious women love and forgive themselves, their food, and their figure.

Marcella leads online and in-person retreats and workshops on mindful eating across the United States. In 2018 she founded the Women, Food, and Forgiveness Academy, a comprehensive online mentorship program to help women heal their struggles with food and body image at the deepest levels of their being.

Marcella's writing can be found in *Elephant Journal, Sivana East, The Tapping Solution Blog, Shambhala Times,* and elsewhere. Her online course, "Lose Emotional and Physical Weight with Tapping," is a top-ten best seller on DailyOM.

Marcella's culinary career began in 1994, when she discovered an escape clause in the rat-race contract and left corporate America to cook for cloistered meditators at Gampo Abbey Buddhist monastery in Cape Breton, Nova Scotia, under the guidance of Pema Chödrön.

From 1994 to 2013, Marcella cooked and taught at meditation retreat centers across North America, including Shambhala Mountain Center, Spirit Rock Meditation Center, and elsewhere.

Marcella certified as a natural foods chef at the Natural Gourmet Institute in New York City in 1998 and taught therapeutic culinary arts at Bauman College in Northern California from 2005 to 2013.

Known for her playful humor, laser-like insight, and deep kindness, Marcella's ability to guide women through their odyssey of transformation comes directly from her own experience of healing the multiple complex traumas of her childhood, combined with more than three decades of Buddhist meditation practice, twenty-plus years in twelve-step recovery, and nearly ten years as a client and practitioner of

Tapping (also called EFT), one of the most outstanding transformational tools ever created.

Marcella is certified in both EFT and Matrix Reimprinting through Tapping the Matrix Academy, founded and run by Rob Nelson in Santa Rosa, California.

Marcella currently lives in the San Luis Valley of Southern Colorado and takes long visits back to her beloved former homeland of Sonoma County, California.